"This is a great read for professionals and non-professionals alike. A book that shows the readers from all walks of life about the WHY, the WHAT and the HOW our minds affect our body inappropriately and vice-versa. Dr. Somera explains in the most simple ways how to prevent and/or remedy those ailments without seeking further treatment from expert professionals."

Dr. Antonio V. Palma, M.D.

———•———

"The book is distinctly intended for lay persons. However, it could be beneficial for the general medical professionals as well, because there are psychological conditions that mimic underlying medical problems and vice versa so that appropriate treatment measures can be undertaken. The author manages to infuse vast body of information into a simple, concise, single volume that explains and recommends sound ways to deal with their own emotional concern."

Dr. E.A. Deloria, Jr., M.D.

———•———

Dr. Angel V. Somera has written and published a thorough and informative collection of weekly articles emphasizing a holistic approach to healing the physical, mental, emotional and spiritual aspects of mental health. This book contains step-by-step instruction, troubleshooting tips for common hurdles, and guidance for treating specific populations. It is an essential tool for any healthcare provider.

K.S. Gavina MSN, RN, CNN QIA

A LAYMAN'S GUIDE TO

COMMON PHYSICAL, MENTAL, EMOTIONAL MALADIES AND THEIR HOME HEALING REMEDIES

Plus...learn about Phobias, Pain, Suffering, Violence, Children's Health and Behavior, the incredible Healing Power of Prayer, and much more

DR. ANGEL V. SOMERA, M.D., F.P.P.A.

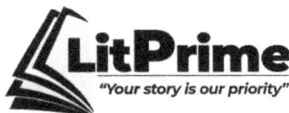

LitPrime
"Your story is our priority"

LitPrime Solutions
21250 Hawthorne Blvd
Suite 500, Torrance, CA 90503
www.litprime.com
Phone: 1-800-981-9893

Published by LitPrime Solutions   03/10/2022

ISBN: 978-1-955944-53-3(sc)
ISBN: 978-1-955944-54-0(e)

Library of Congress Control Number: 2022900395

*To the youth of today in
search for a better lifestyle*

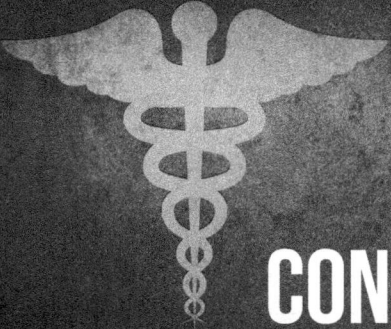

CONTENTS

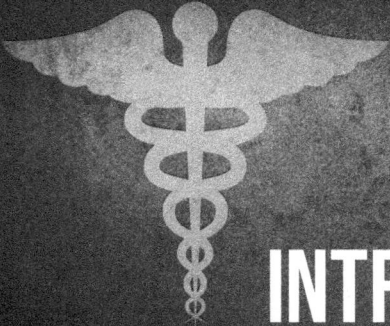

INTRODUCTION

We are living in a time of great change. In these modem times, everyone is seeking for a good and plausible program about health. Health is a life-long process. Studies by health authorities show that the state of health or wellness of every person would greatly depend on his lifestyle. But certainly, we have to consider realistic factors that inevitably affect people's lives. Undeniably, in this new era people are directly or indirectly affected by various stressful changes.

One major threatening factor is our climate change. This is caused by smoke emitted from big factories, and even the burning of sugarcane fields, etc. There are several sources of pollutions in the society: shattering noise, toxic additives from foods, insecticides, water pollutions, junk foods, unbalance diet, alcoholism, drug abuse, etc. Think of the various deadly agents of communicable and infectious diseases–– bacteria, virus, fungus carried and spread by insects (mosquitoes); birds, bats, animals, rabies from dogs, and the traveling man who spreads AIDS, HIV Virus, STD, and his bad habits and criminal behavior-all these and many more destructive activities. Alfred Toffler's "Future Shock" is something to reckon about.

Every human being must have to learn to adjust and adapt to all these dehumanizing situations.

Today, fortunately, the United Nations has come up with a broad and comprehensive concept of health-"WELLNESS". This is defined as a multidimensional state of well-being advocating the existence of positive health in an individual as exemplified by quality of life and a sense of well-being and security.

This book is designed to lend a helping hand and give encouragement to the readers. I incorporate many positive ways to understand and deal with chronic or long-term suffering of human beings. Each part describes the present problems and difficulties with constructive and meaningful solutions to change one's attitude and a positive lifestyle.

As a health-conscious writer, I strongly recommend a "holistic approach" in healing, which basically includes the physical, mental, emotional, and spiritual aspects of man.

All the topics in this book are a compilation of articles I wrote as a columnist for the *Negros Chronicle,* a weekly news publication in the province of Negros Oriental, Philippines. Readers tell me that, they cut the write-ups and keep the clippings for reference on health issues that affect them. Through my brother Ron's vigorous persuasion, I decided to put all the pieces together and publish them into a book. Well, folks, here it is. Hopefully, when you read them, you become aware of the various conflicts that confront you in this life.

Dr. Angel V. Somera

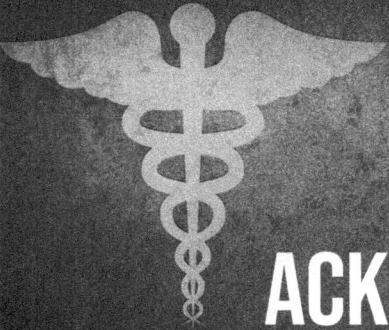

ACKNOWLEDGMENTS

A lot of people are involved in the publication of this book of which I am truly grateful. On top of the list is Ely P. Dejaresco, editor/publisher of the *Negros Chronicle--a* weekly news publication, who gave me his blessings and allowed me to write a column about health issues I am familiar with in my medical profession as a Psychiatrist. The collection of those articles under the heading of "Health is Wealth" is the basis for this book.

I am also indebted to my brother, Veronico "Ron" Somera, who kept reminding me to publish a book version of my column he profoundly believes would be an ideal reference book for people with or without health maladies because it is informative, useful and written in a simple language everybody understands. I trusted Ron who, himself, has authored and produced five successful books: *"Brown American," "Bolo Warriors," "Live Like a Millionaire in the Philippines on $1,500/Month," "Play the Ukulele Like a Pro in Minutes"--all* published in the U.S.A., and *"Buhay Pinoy Overseas"*-a collection of cartoons that depict the lifestyles of Filipinos abroad, published by the prestigious National Bookstore in Manila and sold in the chain of stores it owns throughout the Philippines.

For this laudable project I give my heartfelt thanks to Ron who scrutinized each article and painstakingly sorted them out into parts or categories for easy reference. He also suggested the rather long title of this book and convinced me that it is a common style used by many authors on the subject of health in America who practically splash the front cover of their books with lengthy titles. To my best assistant Tessie, thanks for patiently correcting the English grammar, typing the articles, then bringing them to the encoder and submit them to the Negros Chronicle for the final printing.

Finally, I wish to acknowledge and thank the various authors of the reference books shown at the end of the book for their professional expertise. I also express my profound gratitude to God, the Holy Spirit, for the guidance provided in sharing my own medical experience and expertise into all these articles.

Thank you one and all.

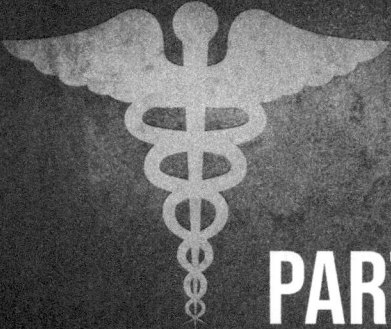

PART I

GENERAL VIEW ON HEALTH, WELLNESS AND BETTER LIVING

Wellness-The New and Broad Concept of Health

As the world turns to a new era, people are inevitably affected by various stressful changes, which Alfred Toffler calls in his famous book as "Future Shock." In order for people to ably survive these extremely difficult and adverse changes, every human being must have to learn to adjust and adapt to these dehumanizing situations.

In the early decades, the prevailing concept of health was confined mostly to the physical-mental aspect. The "mind-body" connection concept ruled on for several decades. This was exemplified by Scott Peck's "The Road Less Traveled," a best seller.

Today, so many stresses lead to the psychosomatic destructions especially to the heart, brain, kidney, and other organ systems of the body. The United Nations come up with a novel and comprehensive concept of "Wellness," a broader health idea. Wellness is defined as "a multidimensional state of well-being describing the existence of positive health in an individual as exemplified by quality of life and a sense of well-being and security."

As an avid advocate **of "holistic healing,"** I strongly believe that in order to heal the body, one must heal the **mind** and the **soul** first.

Here are examples of important dimensions of wellness that must be cultivated by every health-conscious person.

1. **Spiritual Wellness.** This is foremost. This involves the seeking of true meaning and purpose of human existence. "Seek ye first the Kingdom of God..." "What does it profit a man if he gains the whole world but loses the fate of his own soul...!"

2. **Physical Wellness.** This encourages the optimal development of health through the practice of proper health activities for the prevention of diseases.

3. **Mental Wellness.** To cultivate maximally one's mental health through positive thinking and control of bad habits and avoidance of vices.

4. **Emotional Wellness.** This includes the capacity to manage one's feelings, its limitations, and the ability to effectively handle conflicts in life.

5. **Intellectual Wellness.** This encourages potentials life creativity, cultural and other useful human skills for everybody's benefit by reading, learning, and observations.

6. **Social Wellness.** This encourages the interdependence and smooth interpersonal relationships with others in the community.

One has the task of respecting and promoting better communications with others.

7. **Occupational Wellness.** This involves satisfaction and love for work. This is saving enough for one's future, security for his family and his retirement ages.

8. **Environmental Wellness.** This involves the respect and care for the environment and the living things in it. It becomes our prime duty to minimize pollutions and to prevent destructive effects of climate change.

It is very essential to realize the importance of this multidimensional concept of wellness for this is a new way of looking at a person's total health and development as well as to reassure its survival and security existence.

Factors for our Health and for Better Living

The human development of man could be traced on two main factors–– his heredity and his environment. Heredity, as a factor in human development as the saying goes: Nobody can change the color of one's eyes. There are people with blue eyes, while there are also with brown eyes. There are people who are tall, dark and handsome or beautiful, while there are those fair in complexion and short. The descendants' physical features would tell who their ancestors were. In other words, the hereditary predisposition shows that man cannot change whatever genetic endowment he acquires from his ancestors, like the deadly diseases or illnesses (hypertension, diabetes, cancers, heart diseases, etc.).

Environment, as a factor in the human development includes sleep, diet, exercise and recreation. Man's health is precious. It depends on his lifestyle. He should sleep 7 to 8 hours at night; should eat well balanced diet with fruits and vegetables; should exercise regularly to maintain a strong and healthy body; and should recreate or rest to minimize so much stress. And by doing the above-mentioned tips would help prevent whatever hereditary or genetic illnesses or diseases.

It's time to change our lifestyle and bad habits for longer and better living. If symptoms persist, go to the right doctor.

May God bless us all!

Life's Problems

*"The answer to problems
lies in facing them."*
William Barett

Everyone in this world has all kinds of problems, too numerous to mention. No one is spared from this common inheritance and experience. The only difference is that some people are troubled and overwhelmed by their problems, while others are coping and managing them. Some people handle their problem so well that they are mistaken to have no problem at all. They are so efficient.

One of the primary goals of psychotherapy or counseling is to help the troubled individuals manage or resolve their deep-seated conflicts; marital or family or other problems in life that incessantly disturb them. This means that this affected person will fully realize and seriously deal with them realistically and make a good decision and follow through to go on with life courageously.

However, there are individuals who are confused and lose their confidence or easily discouraged. This will undermine their built-in potential for healing or functioning. Unfortunately, some are overwhelmed by their problems, they do not know what to do and become so depressed that they reach the **point of despondency**- feeling of worthlessness, helplessness, and hopelessness-then, commit suicide. This morbid situation is only true to the defeatist and emotionally unstable person.

Effective Solutions to Problems in Life:

- Live simply but comfortably.
- Be a well-organized person.
- Study well the causes of your problems.
- Consult reliable experts to help difficult conflicts to be resolved.
- Develop a spiritual lifestyle: A strong and alive faith. Always pray to the Holy Spirit for any problem in your life. Always thank God for His guidance.

The Secret to a Long Life

> *"To be seventy years young is*
> *far more cheerful and hopeful*
> *than to be forty years old."*
> Oliver W. Holmes

It is an inevitable fact that all of us age and after living for a while we die. Along with age comes the specter of disease, loneliness, mental disability and stresses of life. The perennial question is how can the ravages of time show in our body? It may be something like this–– at age 30 your skin becomes excessively dry and wrinkle; at 40 stiffness and pain in your joints; at 50 high cholesterol and borderline diabetes; at 60 heart disease or osteoporosis.

Studies have shown some basic facts: Exercise delays aging especially in the onset of arthritis and osteoporosis. Authorities claim that low level exercise like taking the stairs instead of the elevator, walking short distances even if for only 10 minutes twice a day could be good.

Staying out of the strong heat of the sun increases wrinkles except the early sunlight at 6 to 8 A.M., which is rich in ergosterol good for absorption of calcium for the bones.

Relaxation and meditation are stress-busters and can prevent disease.

High vegetable diet packed with antioxidants, enzymes and fibers are good for health. Eat high-octane foods like leafy green and red veggies, carrots, broccoli that contains beta carotene (Vitamin A). Avoid smoking, heavy drinking and other bad habits.

Doing crossword puzzles and regular reading can delay and prevent memory loss.

Eating compulsively and obsessively will lead to obesity, diabetes, heart disease and Alzheimer's disease.

Type "A" personalities (pressure-driven individuals) age faster than relaxed ones.

Go fruity, eat fruits like papaya, banana, apples, kiwi, star apple, mangoes, melon which are power-packed nutrient foods. Eat nuts, too for health.

Dehydroepean erosterone (DHEA)-as one grows older, production of this hormone slows down. Go easy on high glycemic foods like white rice, white bread, pastries, pasta, etc.

Avoid saturated fat from animals, which causes high bad cholesterol (LDL) that would result to hypertension, heart disease and stroke.

Pursue and Develop your Potential

Everyone has inside himself a piece
of good news. The good news is that
you really don't know, how good you
can be, what your potential is."

Anne Frank

Everyone born in this world has been created by God for a certain purpose. Undoubtedly, our Creator has given us the basic tools like our brain (intelligence), talents and the opportunities to develop our inherent potentials. It is up to the person to make use of them. Man should wisely use this initiative, <u>Free Will</u> and energy to harness and fulfill his potential being. God respects absolutely this freedom of whether man will do and work sincerely to accomplish his desired ambition or plan of his life. This action that man pursues may either end in success or failure.

Authorities claim that people in the average use only 10% of their creative potential. They do not develop more than the minimum yet they have more resources to attain the maximum. They wish for fulfillment but unfortunately, fail to achieve the challenge of their own power because they lack the basic desire to do better than they should do. They easily give up.

John C. Tomey said, "The secret of becoming a great person is as easy as desiring it. For desire means to wish earnestly, to crave, to yearn, to long for." It is said that <u>wonderment, curiosity, and adventure are the vital motivation of an interesting life</u>. There are so many interesting and meaningful activities and experiences in life which may become a challenge. Man is constantly inspired of learning something new and fulfilling something he could not accomplish before.

<u>Interest and motivation are essential factors in developing one's potential.</u> Interest must come from our desire and active participation. Motivation is a great impetus. It grows gradually until we become obsessed that we will not let a day pass without accomplishing it. Someone said that "Life is not dull; we make it dull only by limiting our potential." Very true indeed.

So let us pursue our beautiful dream--our magnificent obsession until we can fully actualize our full potential in life. Then we realize that "This is what God wants us to be!" Pope John Paul II said, "In God's plan there is no such thing as chance." So, let us fulfill our destiny as what God wants us to be. Manny Pacquiao could have remained a poor boy from Lubao, General Santos, had he not pursued and developed his potential of being the greatest Filipino World Champion Boxer.

Serendipity in Survival

"It isn't that a person is like, it is how
a person interacts with situations
that determines survival."
A.L. Siebert, PhD (Psychologist)

Many of us Filipinos have experienced different kinds

of adversities in life. Undeniably, we have defeatist and fatalistic attitude. We easily give up. Fatalism is a belief that all events are predetermined by fate and therefore, inevitable. A logical solution to this negative attitude is what Dr. Siebert termed as serendipity. This is a positive attitude where a survivor turns a disruptive life event or adversity into a desirable development and thus, preventing himself from becoming a victim. "Survivors are people who look for hope in situations of hopelessness," Siebert says.

Some of us may still remember some worse natural disasters that happened in our country. It's quite amazing, as if an act of miracle has happened, some people still survived amidst extreme catastrophic situations. For instance, the recent collapse of a very deep mining pit in Baguio where several miners perished is one such case. About half a dozen of them still survived without food for several days or almost a week. The rescued miners were interviewed on how they managed to live through the harrowing experience. They said they prayed hard, sipped trickles of rainwater that dripped through the rocky crevices and ate their own clothes. And they never lost hope of being rescued. Another most grueling and brutal situation where thousands of our own soldiers as well as American prisoners of war, survived during the infamous Death March from Bataan to Capas, Tarlac in 1942. Most of the soldiers were starved, exhausted, wounded, sick, bitter and demoralized. They received inhuman treatment from their captors in the prison camps, many prisoners even drank their own urine just to live. Many still survived through the spirit of serendipity.

Dr. Siebert suggests serendipity guidelines as learned from survivors in his research, to wit:

- Learn to welcome adversity or misfortune. Be a

positive thinker. As the saying goes, "When life hands you a lemon, then make a lemonade." Or, "Every dark cloud has a silver lining."

- You may laugh or cry. If you can't laugh, then cry. This calms your emotion and regains emotional stability.
- Be playful and curious. Toy with the passing crisis.
- Get tough and flexible. "When the going gets tough, then get tough going."
- Be optimistic and don't lose hope. Expect a good outcome out of a crisis. "If winter comes, can spring be far behind?"
- Develop empathy skills. Put yourself in other's shoes.
- Take action and be practical. If what you're doing isn't working, then do something else.
- Of course, have strong faith in the Lord, and fervently pray.
- Never forget that miracles do always happen.

The Lesson of Balancing in Life

"There can be no real and abiding happiness without sacrifice."
H.W. Sylvester

In life, people may not truly realize the value of balancing for to them, balancing is only good and advantageous for circus light rope performer who masters the art of balancing as a career for a living.

According to an American writer and psychiatrist, Dr. Scott Peck, in his famous book "The Road Less Travelled" every human being should learn to balance his lifestyle. It is just like a child who likes to learn how to bike but first of all, has to practice balancing with the bicycle. And that in the beginning the inexperienced child will inevitably experience serious falls especially when he tries to negotiate with the sharp curves of the deep and winding road due to lack of balance. He is determined to learn and to continue biking despite the painful and traumatic experience; the sprains, the bruises and the bloody scratches, etc., until he could master maneuvering his bicycle with too much "self-confidence" in him.

According to Scott Peck, balancing is discipline precisely because the act of giving up is painful. In this instance, people in life have been unwilling to suffer the pain of giving up the lesson required to maintain balance. To achieve mastery and success it is imperative to continue relearning the hard lesson throughout our lives. It is painful to give up some of our personality traits, especially the well-established patterns of behavior or even the childish or pleasurable lifestyles if one is to travel very far on the journey of life.

To be able to live peacefully and meaningfully well with others, let us always observe **moderation** in all our activities. This is called the **Virtue of Temperance.** For instance, we must control our appetites to live well and be healthy. We should temper our anger; otherwise we die of hypertension or heart attack.

Always remember the **"Golden Mean"** philosophy.

Reduce the Risk of Disease

All living and responsible health-conscious people must always be aware that everyday, they are waging a war against unseen and silent enemies that are potentially deadly. Doctors call them as foreign invaders and vectors of death-biologically termed as bacteria, viruses, fungi, and parasites. These microscopic elements that can expose the body to cause a disease are found anywhere around us–– in the water, food, animals, insects, and people. All these germs or killers are always ready to march straight into our body by way of contamination or infection. Many of us are not aware of these microscopic battles because we have our immune system that repels or destroys most of the invaders before the onset of symptoms. If our immune system is strong, with its fighter cells (example: B-cells and T-cells, macrophages and antibodies) then, victory is won for our body and no disease would occur! However, if the harmful germs gain the upper hand, you get sick and if your defenses are so weak possibly, you may succumb and die. But if you need to boost your defenses with effective medications (potent antibiotics, sulfas, and other treatments), you will live!

It is too unfortunate that a lot of people are so ignorant and virtually know nothing about the dangers of these extremely harmful organisms.

Studies show that every year, millions of people travel around the world, often transporting disease-causing agents. According to an article in the journal, Clinical Infectious Diseases, "virtually all of the contagious virulent infections" can be spread by international travelers.

Some bacteria have developed resistance to antibiotics. The World Health Organization states that the world is heading towards a post-antibiotic era, in which common infection can kill again!

Civil unrest and poverty often hinder government efforts to control the spread of disease.

Despite these disturbing trends, there is much we can do to protect ourselves and our family. Simple and effective cleanliness habits may be within our reach. For instance, we can still strengthen our defenses:

- Enforce immunization shots to children.
- Proper waste disposal.
- Protect our water from contaminations.
- Be sure that our hands are always clean.
- Limit contact with disease-carrying insects by wearing protective clothing; sleep under treated insect nets; eliminate containers of stagnant water where mosquitos could breed.
- Avoid contact with wild animals. If you are bitten or scratched, wash the wounds thoroughly and seek doctor's advice.
- Avoid contact with body fluids from people, like blood and products to stop the spread of infection like AIDS, HIV, etc.
- If possible, stay at home when you are sick.

Unfortunately, many people lack practical knowledge of how to prevent diseases.

Achieving True Happiness

Undoubtedly, people in this planet Earth are seeking for happiness in a variety of ways. Most mundane people are finding instant happiness in "wine, women, and song" and still others generally find happiness and satisfaction in food, sex, drugs, wealth, power and popularity. However, minority of spirituality-oriented people seek true contentment in their religious belief. Hence, perception of happiness differs greatly in many people depending on their experiences, orientations and motivations.

For instance, Jacqueline Kennedy said, "I am the happiest woman when I'm alone." Og Mandino believes that, "The only source of happiness is within me and I will begin to share it." his saying is true for this was concurred by someone who said: "A joy that's shared is a joy made doubled." Og Mandino aptly said, "There is no happiness in having and getting, but only in giving."

A successful research finding by an American psychologist Dr. Sonja Lyubomirsky, found eight essential steps toward achieving a more satisfying life, which includes the following: (1) Count your blessings. (2) Practice acts of kindness. (3) Savor life's joys. (4) Thank a mentor. (5) Learn to forgive. (6) Invest time and energy with friends and family. (7) Take care of your body (health). (8) Develop strategies for coping with stress and hardships.

As a person with a high emotional quotient (EQ), you must develop your happiness habit by accepting your shortcomings and the harsh realities of life and enhancing your social, intellectual, emotional and spiritual potentials. Happiness is your pristine birthright. So, take it and share it with others.

Follow well the "eight (8) steps" above, and you'll never fail. It's guaranteed!

It's Tough to be Sick

Many people have experienced many forms of sickness; from a mild headache to a more serious ailment like a debilitating flu.

When one is down, the moment when he is really

weakened to the point of being absent from work, he loses his income and reduces nearly to "zero" production.

Here is the Psychiatric explanation:

When a person is really sick, he regresses into an infantile level of adjustment that makes him totally dependent on the people around him, like his family, and the personnel in the hospital, respectively. The hospital becomes a surrogate mother to him.

In order not to be a victim again of the same serious illness, the patient has to fully cooperate with the doctor's order.

It pays to be a healthy conscious person! Always see a doctor for any health problem that you encounter before it's too late.

Positive Lifetime Changes

"Man alone, of all the creatures of the earth can change his own pattern. Man alone is the architect of his own destiny."
Wilford Paterson

Every person with a right attitude or normal mind most often desires to, at least improve his state in life. One of the important behavioral weaknesses that adversely affects human beings are his destructive habits such as smoking, drinking, compulsive gambling, lying (dishonesty), cheating, materialistic and hedonistic pursuit in life, and his lukewarm treatment of his religion, etc. All these bad habits have been acquired in the course of our earthly living.

Bad habits are hard to break for they are acquired conditionally constant and repeated acts or behavior. Hence, they become behavioral pattern which are acted upon unconsciously. Habits are so important in our life. Therefore, the good habits must be reinforced for they affect our eternal destiny.

Definitely, a person who truly manifests a good character must be emulated by all. But a person who lives in a faulty and vicious lifestyle and never changes his behavior is known to be a "sociopath," in Psychiatry. He is already callous to change. No amount of counseling can dent an incorrigible person. These are the criminally-inclined people, like some of our politicians. However, there are also morally good individuals in our society. Only, some are victims of evil schemes of others, like bribery without thinking of the future consequences that would affect them and their families.

"God grant me the serenity to accept the things I cannot change, courage to change the things I can, and the wisdom to know the difference," (Serenity Prayer.)

Healthy Moves on Our Body

Definitely, medical science has made its tremendous progress towards its good health and wellness; conquering infectious and communicable diseases, thus reassuring our health, happiness and much longer lifespan.

It's so interesting to know that advancement in medical researches has discovered healthy moves that have turned our body into a formidable healing machine!

It is now proven that the mind can heal the body by positive thinking. Amazingly, the reverse is also true; the body can heal the mind. For instance, when **endorphins** (positive hormones that cause a sense of well-being) are released through exercises or other forms of positive bodily movements, they give a feeling of well-being and a sense of fulfillment. When you move your body, your blood flows faster and raise your metabolic rate which burns calories and releases hormones that relieve pain and put you in a good mood.

It is a fact that moving your body through exercise, dance, playing musical instruments, moderate working, or whatever this will help your staying well by keeping you limber and fulfilling a sense of satisfaction. When you feel good outside, you also feel good inside within you!

Positive movements also prevents illness by boosting your immune system. It releases tension and stress. Just think how wonderful you feel when you dance! It's a great exhilarating experience!

These healthy moves can do the same positive feeling for everyone. Studies by health and athletic authorities claim that proper movements like controlled exercise or moderate work in any form will consequently benefit the body with the following positive advantages:

- Decrease anxiety and tension
- Manage deadly stress
- Prevent headaches and other bodily pains
- Reduce symptoms of depression
- Improve appearance and posture
- Increase strength and energy levels
- Enhance self-esteem
- Improve mental alertness
- Expand your social life
- Make you feel sexier and younger
- Help you relax and calm
- Improve you mood and feel great
- And definitely, make your quality of life so much better

So let's take good care of our body so that our body will function like a **good healing machine** the way God created it to function!

The Healing Power of Good Emotion

*"A cheerful mind and a healthy body
make a happy man in this world."*
John Locke

A recent TV report claims the Filipinos are the most emotional people in the world. This observation is exemplified and confirmed in our entertainment world where our players profoundly emote laughter and tears in equal passion.

The foremost psychologist William James defines emotion as a state of mind that manifests itself by sensible changes in the body. Psychologists say that a man is emotionally mature if he learns and practices the art of using his positive emotions which makes him genuinely happy and contented. Positive or pleasant emotions will help him in every endeavor of life, work, in his family, in social relations, and in his adjustments in the world at large.

Psychologists classify emotions in tow groups: The pleasant emotions--example: love, joy, hope, courage, equanimity, and agreeableness. Unpleasant emotions--example: anger, hate, fear, discouragement, grief, dissatisfaction, etc.

Our body knows the secret of optimal hormone balance. To be able to do this, we have to provide our body and mind with optimum stimulus of the pleasant or cheerful emotions brought about by endorphins-the "happy hormone." Thus, a happy emotional disposition of mind is needed and should be the central aim in achieving a strong healing power of good emotion.

Here are some effective ways of achieving positive emotions in life. The following are:

- Keep yourself responsive to simple things in life. Don't ask for the unusual things for your pleasurable pursuit. Simply be contended with the wonderful world of colors, sound, smell, and sight around you.
- Avoid watching for any "knock in your vehicle". Neurotic or worrisome people always believe that there is something wrong with their health. Psychiatrists call them as "hypochondriacs".
- Learn to love your work. If a person *dislikes* his work, he still suffer from psychosomatic illness", an emotionally-induced disorder.
- Love people. Be an important part of the community. Get involved in "kapamilya" (family).
- Get the good habit of being a cheerful person. A humorless person often ends up in the doctor's clinic. Happy people seldom get sick and live longer lives.
- Make the present moment an emotional success. This is God's time. Enjoy it! Remember- "Happy people are healthy people!"

Ways to Conquer Frustrations

"My God, my God, why hast thou forsaken me?"

Psalm 22:1, KJV

In life, inevitably rich or poor has experienced frustration in one way or another. We often hear people suffering from extreme despair secondary to utter unrequited love like the Love Story of Shakespeare's Romeo and Juliet, and other sorrowful episodes in life here parents were tortured to death, leaving the helpless children to survive in war, etc. Frustration is synonymous to depression, disappointment, discouragement, despair, failure or defeat. In psychiatry, utter depression means the feeling of **despondency.** This means that the person has finally reached the end of his life-the feeling of worthlessness, the feeling of helplessness, and the feeling of hopelessness. At this point, if there would be no psychiatric help through the use of antidepressant, death is eminent. The depressed patient could commit **suicide** because the patient is deprived of **serotonin-the** mood-elevating neurotransmitter in the system. Before the discovery of this antidepressant medication, scores of depressed individuals who were extremely depressed took their own lives, without exemption including psychiatrists, clergies, ministers, writers and doctors.

However, there are still ways to conquer frustrations in life:

- Be a master of yourself. You must honestly have emotional self-control.
- Always practice strong peaceful thinking.
- Before going to bed, flush out from your mind the bad or negative emotions.
- Turn to Almighty God, our refuge and strength, a tested help in times of trouble. (Psalm 46:1 MB)
- Don't delay before it's too late! Immediately seek for psychiatric help!

Holistic Healing

In my years of psychiatric practice and experience, after my specialization at the U.P.––PGH Medical Center in Manila, I was wholly influenced by a Freudian Concept in the treatment of the mind using basically the concept of the **"unconscious and libido".** But today my paradigm shift has totally turned to the **mind-spiritual dimension.** I found out that this is the most relevant approach to the effective healing of the conflicted mind and troubled soul. Hence, the successful holistic healing.

As a psychotherapist, I am a strong believer that in order to fully heal the body of the person, his mind and soul has also to be healed.

Man must realize that when he commits sin it would affect his whole being-mentally, emotionally, and spiritually. He would suffer mental torture. The healing is that he has acknowledge his sin, be sorry for it, and to reconcile with God by promising not to sin again, and to do some mortification or penance in order to be free again.

Here is a beautiful Message of Salvation for the repentant soul...A man May Go to Heaven--

Without health,
Without wealth,
Without fame,
Without a great name,
Without learning,
Without culture,
Without beauty,
Without friends,
Without 10,000 other things

But he can never go to Heaven without CHRIST!!!

Jesus answered, "I am the Way, the Truth, the Life. No one comes to the Father except through Me." (John 11:6, ESV)

Meaningful Reflections from Desiderata:

"Poetry is the record of the best and happiest moments of the best minds."
Percy B. Shelley

"Desiderata" is an old but famous free verse poem written by an unknown writer from an ancient world. This writer must be a man of letters. His writing has a great foresight for its relevance transcended not only during his time but for several generations until today.

The word "desiderata" simply means goals, aims, or purposes. The insightful author has a paramount objective in guiding people's lives especially during times of confusions and crisis. He mainly suggested sound tenets to be followed well before one could achieve peace and happiness in this world. He wisely counsel: "Go placidly (Be calm and relax for this will prevent hypertension, heart attack or stroke.)...Amid the noise and haste-remember, what peace there may be in silence." (Strive to live in a quiet and tranquil environment away from chaos and turmoils.)

- "Search for the truth quietly and clearly." Always be honest. The truth will set you free.
- "Listen to others even to the dull and ignorant." They too have their story to tell. You must not ignore the uneducated. They are your brothers. Listen to them. You also need them.
- "Avoid loud and aggressive people." They are vexations to the spirit. Avoid the loud mouths,

the evil or criminally inclined. They are so irritating and destructive.

- "Take kindly the counsel of the years." Listen to the good advices of the experienced and wise persons.
- "Always be at peace with GOD." God is our refuge and Savior. Always pray and thank Him for all your blessings.
- "Remember, with all the sham, drudgery and broken dreams it is still a beautiful world. (In spite of the hypocrisy, corruption and unfulfilled ambition, it is still a wonderful planet.)

Mental Defense Mechanisms-Contrive Alibi

*"These adaptive processes are
tricky psychological (cover-up)
maneuvers that allow the sinner
to emerge as a good guy."*

Let us continue to reveal more interesting psychological defense maneuvers used by people to cope up with the unrelenting conflicts and stresses in life.

Here are more of them:

- **Intellectualization.** A maneuver used by person of average intelligence to cover up their hidden inadequacies or inferiority complex. They talk big on their accomplishments, shows diplomas, certificates, official ranks, memberships of organizations, travels, and drop names (connections) just to impress others and prop up their weak egos.
- **Rationalization.** One does something and

invents a seemingly logical explanation or reason for the action that was made. A rejected guy whose girlfriend left him, may say-"Well, she is not my type." (A sour grape or sweet lemon attitude.)

- **Nomadism.** The continual wandering from place to place. The person who frequently change his residence, jobs, or even his partners in life.
- **Displacement.** A feeling is transferred from its actual object to a substitute. An original feeling of hostility towards one's parents is transferred to other authority figures.
- **Compensation.** An attempt to disguise the presence of a weak or undesirable trait by emphasizing a desirable one. Example: A person who is physically unattractive may attempt to gain popularity by developing a charming manner and a good conversationalist.
- **Overcompensation.** This is a pathological defense exemplified by persons who are show-offs, loudmouths, etc. who irritate people when they are around.
- **Undoing.** People who make up for hurting a friend. The individual divests himself of painful feeling (i.e. guilt) by doing a repetitive cleansing ritual in the hope of relieving anxiety. Example: The washing mania of Lady Macbeth for the murder of Macdoff.
- **Symbolization.** An object or idea is used to represent another idea or object. Example: An elongated object like a knife may represent a phallic symbol, and a strawberry or a red flower

may represent female genitalia. A ship, ocean or mothering figure may represent the mother.

- **Fixation.** The arrest of maturation at any immature level of psychosexual development. Example: Presence of enuresis into adolescence. Thumb sucking behavior, or schizophrenia-a total regression to infantilism.
- **Conversation** (Or Somatization). This mechanism allows a person to cover up a negative feeling to be channeled to a physical symptom. Example: A psychological paralysis of a limb (arm) which prevents its use for aggressive purposes (striking, boxing, killing, etc.)
- **Restitution.** A defense mechanism devised by a single person to relieve his mind of a load of guilt by restitutive acts (reparations). It may become the motive of life. Example: A former ill-repute woman who lived in the house of prostitution. She left and started to faithfully serve a church congregation until she died of old age.

As true Christians, we cannot always live using these defense mechanisms as cover-up which hid the truth. Truth is essential to healing. Hence, to discover the truth, we truly need to seek professional assistance to finally ease the relentless pains of anxiety and serious illnesses which bring the untold miseries and shortens our lives.

Drug and Substance Dependence-- The Modern Scourge of Man

Psychologists and social scientists throughout the world

have been studying and researching feasible causes of drug and other substance abuse. Experts on the subject have come up with the various etiological causes of why man resorts to abuse prohibited substances and drugs when they know that it's harmful that can even lead to death.

There are **Probable Concepts** that would explain why people take prohibited drugs and substances.

A. **The Sigmund Freud's Life Theory and Death Theory.** Consciously, man always strive to live and be healthy by eating good and nutritious food, having proper exercise, rest and good sleep, etc. This is known as **Life Theory.** But unconsciously, there is another instinctual drive that would lead man to his own death-life excessive drinking, smoking, and overindulgence in anything. This is **Death Theory.**

B. **Pharmacologic Theory.** This is the tendency for a drug or substance to stimulate drive to alter perception and to produce euphoria (sense of well-being). This is the most significant mechanism of action addicts like.

C. **Psychodynamic Hypothesis.** States that drug abusers are suffering from mental and emotional trauma during their childhood or formative years which are deeply unresolved. The use of drugs or substances helps them alleviate temporarily these unpleasant conflicts.

D. **The Learning Theory (Behavioral).** States that the conditioning of drug taking behavior is believed to immediately relieve tension, and engender the feeling of euphoria, not knowing the detrimental effects of drugs.

The Characteristic Traits of a Drug or Substance Dependent: Immature, irresponsible, lazy, too dependent, pleasure-seeker, pathological liar or sociopath, rebellious, inadequate or inferior, oversensitive, hostile, lacks respect for law and order, and without spiritual values.

Possible Factors that contribute to a drug and substance dependency: Broken family, overprotective family-spoiling the child (palangga system), chaotic family, and peer group pressure (barkada system), poor and permissive environment, bad influence of Rock Stars and other indecent personalities through Mass Media, etc.

The Remedial Solution to minimize this Social Problem. There should be cooperation, concerted and relentless efforts of the concerned parents, school, church, and community. There should be strict implementation of the Drug Laws.

So help us God from this evil menace.

Preventive Lifesavers

"An ounce of prevention is
worth a pound of cure."
Old Proverb

How many precious lives have been lost because people failed to head a sound health advice or were unable to recognize or identify early signs and symptoms of diseases? It's a pity because of pure ignorance. Many of our people see the doctor only when they already feel very bad, not knowing that at this stage the disease must have already set in the body and has become difficult to treat or cure.

The problem is that people just ignore or procrastinate consulting the doctor. This is a plain "manana habit." People are very stubborn indeed and never learn the good dictum-"Prevention is better than cure." Most people would just philosophize when they cannot do anything about the situation and will only say, "We all die anyway." This is a statement that reflects a fatalistic attitude-"Consuelo de bobo" type of flimsy rationalization. It is very ironic that during these times, when most people have learned a lot of vital information on health matters from the mass media and other segments of society, there is no reason why they still shun early medical consultations. Medical specialists share significant health advices that remind and warn clients the importance of preventing the occurrence of serious diseases. Let us mention some of these common serious diseases that can be easily prevented.

- How many people get early bone fracture because of osteoporosis? Why? Because young people take soft drinks (soda) instead of buying milk (a difference of a few pesos) or take other calcium-rich foods during the bone-building years of adolescence and early adulthood. A regular exercise like brisk walking (aerobics) can also help prevent osteoporosis. Women should take estrogen for the first five years after they menopause, a period when most bone weakening occurs.
- Another common preventable killer disease is smoking. A strong warning sign: "Stop smoking before it kills you!" Studies and statistics have definitely proven that smoking is extremely harmful to your lungs, heart, throat, stomach and highly predisposes one to cancer because

of a carcinogenic substance-nicotine. It could adversely affect other non-smokers in the family known as "passive smokers."

- This is very important. Be aware of your family medical background. For instance, if there is a positive history of cancer in your family, then, you have a possibility of strong genetic tendency-a hereditary predisposition. You inherit the familial disease.

Well, there are still many early signs and symptoms of fatal ailments that could still be prevented and be remedied if discovered much earlier. Many have been saved because of this early detection.

Here are some sound preventive measures:

1. Have a regular medical (physical) and complete laboratory checkup especially when you reach 30 years and above (most degenerative diseases start here).
2. Watch what you eat. i.e. a lot of fresh vegetables, fruits and a balanced diet. Avoid too much fat, salt and sugar.
3. Do a regular (aerobic) exercise daily or 3 times a week to strengthen your cardiovascular and immune systems.
4. Know the principles of "Stress management" and apply them strictly in your life.
5. Most of all-Live a well-balanced lifestyle and a Christ-centered life!

These are all wise reminders to achieve ultimate health, genuine happiness, and a much longer life span. Guaranteed, my friends!

Plan for a Healthier and Longer Life

*"Life, if lived correctly, will bring forth
health and long life. If abused, it will
bring forth illness and early death."*
Anonymous

As we go through another year, scientific studies have consequently shown that the outcome of whether a person will live better and much longer or not at all will depend on the following essential factors that health authorities and doctors highly recommend for a healthier, longer and happier life on earth.

1. **Realize that a longer life is chiefly up to you.** Barring accidents, practically all known diseases of man are preventable. Therefore, longevity is up to the individual concern. He must be a highly health-conscious person. "An ounce of prevention is worth a pound of cure."
2. **Have a periodic medical check-up.** Chest x-ray may reveal an early lesion, a prostate exam cancer; the cardiogram may indicate an arteriosclerosis, chemical blood analysis may show abnormal findings, a blood pressure reading, hypertension, etc.
3. **Don't ignore early symptoms.** For example, a recurrent headache and dizziness may indicate a space-occupying lesion in the brain; an aneurysm may manifest a severe dissecting pain over the chest, etc. Know the early signs of cancer.
4. Shorten one's life. Avoid junk foods. Load on fruits and vegetables. Eat moderately

and take essential vitamins and minerals as supplements.

5. Have a good sleep, rest, relaxation and worthwhile vacation with your family.
6. Stop smoking for it's very bad for one's health.
7. Watch out for alcohol. It carries a lot of calories and causes cirrhosis of the liver and causes early death.
8. Regular exercise is a must. It is very beneficial for the whole body for it prolongs life.
9. Be optimistic and have a sense of humor. "A merry heart does good like a good medicine, but a broken spirit dries up the bones." (Gospel)
10. Know how to manage stress. Seek early professional help before it's too late.
11. Develop your true spirituality. This is foremost. Be a God-fearing, a loving and prayerful person. Live a strong virtuous life, an authentic Christian. Strong faith hastens healing!

Our Split Brain

> *"The first step to knowledge is to know that we are ignorant."*
>
> Cecil

Modem Psychology report reveals a very interesting finding that we have a "split brain"-the left and the right brain with a specific function. This actually refers to our left and right hemispheres.

Neurosurgeons in the U.S.A. accidentally operated on a girl named Victoria who got sick both with measles and scarlet fever. She started to have uncontrollable seizures, which were controlled by anticonvulsant drugs for a while, but later recurred. So the neurosurgeons operated on her head by cutting the Corpus Callosum that connected the left and the right hemispheres which stopped the terrible convulsions (the function of the Corpus Callosum is it allows the information to pass back and forth between the hemispheres).

The functions of the hemispheres...each hemisphere has a special task.

1. The Left Hemisphere:
    a. Verbal-It is programmed for language-related skills: speaking, understanding language, carry on a conversation, reading, writing, and spelling.
    b. Mathematical Skills-Adding, subtracting, multiplying, dividing, and solving complex problems in calculus, physics and so on. Generally, the right hemisphere can perform simple addition and subtraction but not more than complex mathematics.
    c. Analytic-It processes information by analyzing each separate piece that makes up a whole.
2. The Right Hemisphere:
    a. Nonverbal-It is mute. It has a child-like ability to read, write and understand speech like understanding simple sentences and read simple words.
    b. Spatial-It is programmed to solve spatial problems such as arranging blocks to match a geometric design. It is best in arranging blocks (both the left and the right hemispheres combined).
    c. Holistic-It processes information by combining parts into a meaningful whole.

It is involved in recognizing and producing emotional expressions.

Are you a "left-handed" or a "right-handed" person? Generally, analysts say that one is a right-brained individual if he is creative, intuitive, and artistic. You are left-brained if you are reasonable, logical and rational. Studies have shown that our brain gets improved as we use it, and loses its function if we don't use it at all.

The Defective Human Brain

"All men are liable to error..."
John Lock

According to scientific anthropological findings our human brain is still undergoing gradual evolutionary changes. Hence, man, in many of his activities and behavior is never perfect. So, we have to understand why we deal so poorly with the demands of our world. Consider the following timetable:

- 3,000,000 years ago, hominids bid goodbye to the apes.
- 2,000,000 years ago, first tools were created.
- 60,000 years ago, first flowers were found in graves.
- 40,000 years ago, first use of fire.
- 35,000 years ago, modem man appeared and language evolved.
- 13,000 years ago, grain was ground.
- 10,000 years ago, last ice age ended.
- 9,500 years ago, first complicated settlement.

- 7,000 years ago, early switch from hunting and gathering to agriculture.
- 6,500 years ago, the Old Kingdom of Egypt.

With these important findings now we can fully understand that the immediate cause of our destructiveness in this life is the gross in efficiency the human brain. We were basically taught that our brain is a marvel of complexity, the billions of cells serving such functions as rational thought, emotion, coordination and perception. But we have to understand that because of its continuing development, it has not been fully developed yet and therefore, we still expect deficiencies in its functions. We might tolerate such minor deficiencies like mistakes, poor memory, slip of the tongue, forgetfulness, etc., but the gross humanities like war, cruelties, the slaughter of millions of innocent people, failures of marriages, dishonesties, corruptions, frequency of suicides, etc. explain why the brain is still defective in its functions. It is not a perfect or reliable organ.

Men always argue. They do not have the same or identical views. They might agree on the same idea, but with different opinions (opinions are not facts).

People have different beliefs and ideological system because of various traditions, cultures, and religions that influence their behavior. For instance, St. Thomas More, the English Statesman, author of **UTOPIA** an imaginary description of an idealistic or perfect state which never existed. But St. Agustin wrote a more realistic book **TRUE CONFESSION** explaining why man commits sin because of his human pleasurable carnal desires.

The above factual discovery proves that our brain is defective because it is still in the process of development. This is the reason why we never find peace, harmony, perfect human relations in this worldwide existence. Probably, this must be the reasons why God the Father sends His only Son Jesus Christ to this imperfect and sinful world to save mankind from total destruction.

Reflexology

> *"Modern man seeks healing processes through Conventional and Alternative Medicine."*
>
> Anonymous

Today our folks are submitting themselves to a kind of alternative medicine through the use of the art-the "healing hands" known as "reflexology".

Reflexology is basically from the age-old Oriental Meridian (lines) theory or pathways carrying energy through the body. It uses fingers to exert pressure on reflex zones or specific points located on the feet that correspond to different parts and systems of the human body. For example, applying pressure to a point on your big toe will stimulate the flow of energy to your head and sinusis and may help them up. Reflexology works very well on the feet.

Reflexology can be both stimulating and relaxing. It is believed to promote better health through stress-reduction and circulation. It also helps eliminate toxins and balances the body's energy flow.

Reflexologists use it to treat conditions such as asthma, backaches, constipation, headaches, kidney stones, migraines and sinusitis. Practitioners claim that reflexology can also relieve ailments such as acne, cirrhosis of the liver, colds, fatigue, impotence, infections and stress. It is highly recommended for people with anxiety, tension or what is known as "psychosomatic disorders".

The effects of reflexology:

- It releases pain-blocking endorphins into the blood stream.
- It relaxes the body, dilates or widens any constricted blood vessel and improves blood circulation.
- Tips of fingers emit "Kernian Energy" for the healing process.
- Breaks up congestion caused by uric acid and other chemical crystallization in the body.

Precaution: Avoid reflexology to patients who have varicose veins, thrombosis, phlebitis, or ulceration of the foot. And those persons who just underwent major surgery will have to wait for a year or two before reflexology can be applied.

Defense Mechanism

In these modem times, people are living in a world of various conflicts and stresses. Psychologists claim that these adverse factors are the definite causes of mental, emotional, as well as psychosomatic disorders—like hypertension, heart attack, stroke, ulcers, etc. that shorten man's life. How do we cope these terrifying illnesses?

Authorities have discovered a number of psychological processes known as defense mechanism that could be used by patients to be able to manage the above maladies.

Defense mechanisms are specific, unconscious,

intrapsychic adjustments that come into play to resolve emotional conflict and reduce the individual's anxiety. In psychoanalysis defense mechanism is an unconscious resolution of a conflict, whereby the ego is somewhat protected from anxieties.

Common defenses of man:

1. Repression, 2. Suppression, 3. Regression, 4. Fixation, 5. Identification, 6. Incorporation, 7. Introjection, 8. Projection, 9. Rationalization, 10. Intellectualization, 11. Compensation, 12. Reaction formation, 13. Sublimation, 14. Denial, 15. Substitution, 16. Restitution, 17. Displacement, 18. Isolation, 19. Undoing, 20. Dissociation, 21. Symbolization, 22. Idealization, 23. Fantasy.

Conclusion: Defense mechanisms are useful only if used sparingly. Overusing defense mechanism is considered abnormal or what the psychiatrists call "neurotic."

Unraveling Man's Nature

"God gives us men. A time like these demands strong minds, great hearts, true faith, and ready hands. Men who have honor, men who cannot lie."

I.G. Holland

One of the meaningful inquiries in life is-"Who is man?" Shakespeare has a beautiful answer. "Man is the paragon of animals." The Holy Bible represents the Evangelists by animals-a Lion, an Eagle, an Ox, etc. People have caricatured their spouses as for instance-"My wife is a tiger" or, "My husband is a snake." etc.

Now, let us analyze this creature called "man." Modem psychologists dichotomize man into three (3) different components...they call ego states. Sigmund Freud terms them as **ID, EGO, and Superego.** They simply mean as the **CHILD, the ADULT and the PARENTS** in us.

The first personality component is the "ID, or the CHILD" in us. As we know the natural behavior of a child is unbridled or uncontrollable. It is instinctual that children are impulsive. They are too dependent on their mother's care. In the vernacular they only do the **K.K.K. as kaon** (eat), **katulog** (sleep), **kalibang** (defecate). So, it is essential that the mother should know the importance of **mothering.** Otherwise the child will grow abnormally in this world.

The second personality component is the "Adult or Ego State". This is acquired through consistent parental toilet training, reward and punishment, value formation, schooling, peer group interaction and spiritual formation. The child learns the various defense mechanisms and adjustments to his environment. All these values are integrated to his personality and self-fulfilled as a good person in the society.

The third component of his personality is the "Parental or Superego" development. This is the morality or conscience formation. The child will know what is right and what is wrong. He should obey the Commandments and Laws of the Land. This is part of our conscience that makes us guilty or not guilty. Sociopaths or criminals have impaired superego development.

Man must integrate these three components to be a true citizen in this world. Otherwise he will fail to become a good person but a ferocious beast like Hitler!

Infatuation and True Love

Today, majority of our people are confused between

what is real love from mere infatuation which is physical or sexual attraction. Hence, broken marriages result especially to the young and immature couples.

The basic meaning of love according to the psycho-social scientists: Jove is complex yet basically unified emotion comprising the element of tenderness, affection, as well as the feeling of empathy, pleasure in actively devoting thought, energy, time and all other resources, and full acceptance of the uniqueness and individuality of the loved one.

The book, "The Art of Loving" authored by Eric Fromm-a psychoanalyst, describes five major types of love relationships:

1. Brotherly Love--oriented towards all fellowmen
2. Parental Love-towards parents
3. Erotic Love-towards married lovers
4. Self-Love-towards self-own acceptance and self-esteem
5. Love of God-man's need to overcome separateness and to achieve union with his Creator

Psychologists' studies have shown that the ability to give as well as to accept love can develop only if it is nourished by both truly mature and responsible lovers.

The difference between true love and infatuation. According to an American psycho-social scientist, H.A. Bowman: Infatuation may come suddenly but true love takes time to grow. Infatuation may be based on one or two traits (usually on physical attributes-- example beauty and sex appeal), but true love is based on many traits, example character, integrity, industry, responsibility, etc. in infatuation, the person is in love with another person geared for self-gratification, but in true love, there is a feeling of self-fulfillment and identity. ("I want her to be the proud mother of my children.) In infatuation, one feels so insecure all the time, but in real love you work and plan to please the other person till death do you part. In infatuation, you change quickly but in true love it lasts and never dies. It is a lasting commitment and union between two devoted and faithful lovers blessed by God Almighty.

However, unfortunate couples whose marriages are extremely miserable because of serious personality incompatibility can still avail of Judicious Court Settlement under the Family Code of the Philippines that will grant them annulment proving their psychological capacity or incapacity.

Ways to Prevent RAPE

"An ounce of prevention is
worth a pound of cure."
Old Proverb

Recently, a 14-year old girl from Dumaguete City was reported to have been raped by a tricycle driver in broad daylight. The heinous crime has created a frightening signal to our young girls who love to gallivant in our city streets.

Rape is a violent crime with a medical, psychological, legal and social implications. Rape is more than a sexual act. It is an act of aggression and hostility. The word "rape" is derived from the Latin word *"repere"*, meaning "to steal, seize, or to carry away." Authorities define rape as an act of forced sexual intercourse with a female committed against her will by a rapist.

Studies claim that most rapists appear "normal" in

appearance. Potential rapists in society are drug abusers, alcoholics, criminally inclined persons or "sociopaths" and quiet guys who hate women.

Research shows that potential victims of rape are the young girls whose built tends to be plump or "fleshy", innocent or helpless-looking with or without sex appeal.

Here are some effective suggestions that may save girls from being raped:

- Remember, every woman is a potential victim of rape when opportunity allows.
- If possible, do not walk alone at night without any responsible male or female companion.
- Avoid walking along dark, narrow, and isolated places. Always stay at the middle of a well-lighted street where there are people. It's safer.
- If you notice that you are being followed, change direction immediately and run away while there is still time.
- Never entertain any stranger who wants to talk to you. You'll never know his evil intention.
- Avoid looking very sexy or seductive (e.g. wearing shorts, spaghetti shoulder straps, scanty and shapely clothes, dark lipstick, strong perfume and walking life a tiger, etc.).
- If you are staying alone in a house, be sure to double-lock your door to bar any intruder to enter. Do not let any "friendly" male to enter until you absolutely identify him well.
- If the man has a weapon (e.g. with a knife or a gun) just stay calm and pray. Fear can immobilize you. Don't offer any resistance, for to resist, or fight back may result to serious injury or death.
- However, if the rapist is unarmed and you think

you can overcome him because you rely on your self-defense, then, you may fight back just to resist and distract, enough for you to run away and shout for help. A good defense and offense–– <u>Hit his eyes with your finger to blind</u> him.

- Pray to St. Michael Archangel (the Protector) for help.

Cause of Marriage Failure: Money, Sex, and Communication

Money, sex, and communication are frequently cited as the most common reasons for a marriage failure. The following discussion details some of the reasons these three topics are the top contenders for marriage failure, what can be done to avoid these issues, and how a marriage can be restored after suffering from these issues.

Income levels can create difficulty in marriage. Low-income families may be greater affected than middle or high-level income families. Low-income families may not have the resources to take care of basic needs, e.g. medical costs, nutritional foods, housing, etc.

This may lead to increase stress within the relationship, which can lead to increase marital discord, fighting, and ultimately may lead to dissolution of the marriage. Middle and high-income marriages may fight over spending levels, who is earning more/less money, the authority to spend the money, and whether each partner is doing his/her share.

Women, in today's society, are at less financial risk than ever before. As a result, many women expect men to help with the traditional household chores. Since many men still believe this to be woman's work, the equal partnership with both partners bringing in an income, can create problems that are essentially created by money.

Marks of a Happy Marriage

"The sweetest joy, the wildest woe is love."
Baily

Love is the breath of life and the most essential of all human emotions. God created man to love and be loved. It is man's basic need like air, food and water. How tragic that people abuse and lose the magic and love-light glowing in their married life.

Here are suggestions that help couples achieve a long term happiness and satisfaction in their marriage:

1. Start the day with a happy disposition. Have a hearty breakfast together. Whisper to her, "I love you, sweetheart." Kiss the back of her neck tenderly. She loves it. Kiss her again when you return from work, no matter how tired you are.

2. Strive to grow up together as a full human being. Inspire each other to become the best person he/she can be. Compliment and strengthen each other's weakness. Totally accept each other and be tolerant of each other's mistake. Say "I am sorry dear." Love your spouse despite his/her imperfections and faults.

3. If you have an argument, respect your wife's opinion, listen sympathetically and discuss it calmly. Avoid being emotional. Communicate

reasonably well. Don't shout at each other unless there's fire!

4. Avoid keeping secrets or hidden agenda. Be completely open and honest. This will help keep your love alive, encourage faith and builds trust for each other.

5. Don't be unreasonably jealous when your husband is watching the opposite sex. As Bishop Fulton Sheen said, "Looking at a merchandize doesn't necessarily mean intent to buy." Trust each other and don't question his/her fidelity.

6. Plan, discuss your mission, and project or goal intelligently. Share your finance together. Monetary problems may cause marital split-ups.

7. Be trusting and forgiving. Settle your differences in a rational way. Solve your arguments and reconcile before the day ends. Don't bring your problems in bed.

8. Remember birthdays and anniversaries. Be concerned and supportive with each other. This is a tangible sign of love. Make each other happy despite crisis that may happen in life. Always give a meaningful gift for each other-a rose, chocolate, gold necklace, etc.

9. Make an effort to get away from the drudgery of life. Have a candlelight dinner in a specialty restaurant, escape to an out-of-town resort, take a pilgrimage, etc. Leave your cares behind and find a paradise where you enjoy alone together.

10. Have a great sense of humor. Share jokes and funny anecdotes with each other. Always

view life from a positive angle. Remember the saying "Laugh and the whole world will laugh with you. Cry and you cry alone."

11. When you are in public, don't be ashamed to show your affection. Touch and hold hands together. But don't show embarrassing behavior.

12. Make him/her feel that he/she is needed and an indispensable person in your life. You are meant for each other until your hair turns white. This is your loving commitment until the end of our life.

God bless and guide you.

The Importance of Fibers in our Diet

A lot of people must have heard about edible fibers but many do not realize the benefits that they give to our body. A diet high in fibers is undeniably good for our health.

Studies have shown that high-fiber diet helps:

- Prevent and relieve bowel disturbance such as constipation, hemorrhoids, diverticular disease, and irritable bowel syndrome.
- Reduce cholesterol level in the blood.
- Reduce the risk of heart disease.
- Reduce the risk of developing certain types of colon cancer.
- Reduce the risk of diabetes.

Here are some ways to help increase your fiber intake in your diet.

- Switch from white rice and pasta to brown rice and whole wheat pasta.
- Choose breakfast cereals with lots of oats and brans.
- Take at least five servings of vegetables and two servings of fruits every day.
- For healthy snack, go for nuts instead of chips or chocolate.
- Doctors prescribe **"C-lium Fibre"-a** natural soluble fiber preparation to be taken during breakfast. Please follow strictly instructions in the brochure.
- Consult an Internist in case of obstinate constipation.
- Remember that all stool softeners are habit forming when taken regularly.

Holistic Therapy for Optimum Health

1. Promote good Smooth Interpersonal Relationships (S.I.R.) to foster peace and friendship.
2. Appreciate the value of work and shun workaholism as mostly done by Type "A" personalities who are at high risk of stroke or heart attack.
3. Engage in wholesome hobbies and develop your God-given artistic sense and creative talents.
4. Do things in moderation (temperance) at all times. This is the "Golden mean" of life.
5. Manage your time well for this is the secret of pure productivity and success.

6. Adopt a well-balanced lifestyle to add more years to life and life to years.
7. Seek early professional help for any unresolved problem before it becomes helpless and hopeless.
8. You may consider the proven efficacy of known "Alternative Medicine" (i.e. Dietary Supplements, Herbal Remedies, Massage Therapy, Reflexology, etc.) only after consulting your doctor for your medical condition.
9. Have a regular medical checkup to stay healthy and prevent any early-onset illness to take root.
10. But most important at all, be wise and be a real spiritual person–– a true Christian.

Achieving a Balanced Lifestyle

It cannot be denied that when the year is ending, there is also an equal feeling of anticipation of the coming of another new year, especially for people who are always conscious of their respective lifestyles and their respective pursuits in life. And we notice, year in and year out, that people's consciousness is more on health lifestyle.

An experience one has told that he almost died of Acute Pancreatitis *(bangungut)* after attending a fiesta where he ate and drank a lot. Another experience-he was rushed to the hospital due to a "heart attack" and he nearly died.

We have to fully realize that we are living in an "Age of Anxiety" (stress). There are several factors that cause the development of anxiety and tension that inevitably would trigger detrimental distress, recurrent diseases and early death.

Psychiatrists listed positive factors that contribute to the development of constant anxiety and tension in life.

Here is a checklist of factors that would cause health or ill-health in one's life.

1. Are you a smoker or a drinker?
2. Do you eat 3 balanced meals a day?
3. Are you within 5 pounds of your ideal weight?
4. Do you exercise at least 20 minutes, 3 times a week?
5. Do you sleep 7 to 8 hours at night?
6. Do you have several close friends whom you seek/talk regularly?
7. Do you have indoor or outdoor hobbies that you often enjoy?
8. Are you confident of your professional or social abilities?
9. Do you enjoy listening to soothing music and clean jokes?
10. Do you recreate and spend vacation with your family?
11. Are you familiar with relaxation and stress management?
12. Do you not hesitate to seek for professional help if needed?
13. Do you do things in moderation?
14. Are you contented with living a simple life?
15. Are you a God-fearing person and living a truly spiritual life?

Fulfill these major health dictums! Live long and be happy!

When Do You Call a Doctor?

A lot of people are in a dilemma of whether or not they will call a doctor for their problematic symptom. More often than most family members usually decide to wait and observe if the symptoms like fever or pain will be relieved when the first usual or common home remedy is given. But when the initial treatment given failed to relieve the symptoms and observed to be getting worse or it recurs, despite the initial treatment then it could be a sign that the illness is different. And if it is not treated well professionally, it could become worst and serious, and difficult to manage. If complication sets in, it might even cause the early death of the patient. This is the result of the delayed referral to a doctor.

A good lesson of medical ignorance to think about is once a young boy, who after working hard in their farm, got wet in the rain that day and developed terrible colds. The family gave him an anti-cold tablet that late afternoon. But he developed chills and high fever that night. His poor Resistance gave way. The family could not bring him to the emergency hospital for proper treatment. He died of acute culminating pneumonia.

Deciding whether to consult a doctor or not when a member of the family is sick, is a responsibility that should not be taken lightly. More often than not, we are reluctant to consult a doctor because the symptoms or signs are serious enough to warrant the needed service of a doctor.

There are some good rules to follow in referring to a doctor.

1. Any unusual or unexplained condition of the body changes.
2. If the illness persists or last for a long time.

3. If the illness recurs or get worse after the usual treatment.
4. Refer the patient to a doctor when he is not very ill yet. If the illness appears repeatedly.
5. A sudden high fever without apparent cause.
6. Any aches or pain that cannot be explained.
7. Any mental or emotional disturbance like serious constant anxiety, fear, depression, persistent insomnia may be a start of a serious disorder.

A symptom is not a disease...it is a sign of an illness. Remember: "An ounce of prevention is worth a pound of cure."

The Healing Power of Music

*"Music hath charms that soothe
the savage's breast..."*
William Congreve

A lot of people do not realize that a good music has a powerful therapeutic effect in our nervous system. Studies show that selected music is being used in many psychiatric centers in the U.S.A. as well as in Europe as a therapeutic modality. For instance, in hospital wards were depressed patients are confined and exposed to listen to lively, sweet and lilting music have resulted to a high therapeutic response in the patients' behavior, plus a significant early recovery and early discharge rate. The very aggressive and boisterous patients are confined in a ward where they can listen to soft, melodious and relaxing music, thus resulting in the early calming effect of the agitated and violent patients' behavior. Amazingly, the patients become so docile and friendly!

The music therapy made the patients recall the songs that their mothers or love ones used to sing when they were still in their homes, respectively.

"Music has charm that sooths the savage's breast."

A true story of an American soldier who raided a German Camp. One night he spotted a German guard in his post guarding the museum of the camp. While nearing the post where the guard was sited, the American soldier heard a familiar music-"Silent Night" that was played by the German guard with his harmonica. Instead of shooting the guard, the American soldier withdrew and spared the guard from his untimely death.

Music has an important role in our lives, so much so that a certain Rural Health Nurse was madly in love with an ordinary guy who used to serenade her with his good voice. And in return she gave her yes to him by marrying him!

Undoubtedly, one of the inspiring factors that the President elect Duterte used during the last election was his recitation of a Patriotic Song-"I Love the Philippines..." This song is greatly motivating!

Great Lessons of Love

"Take away love and our earth is a tomb."
Robert Browning

During "Valentine's Day" we focus ourselves on the beautiful thoughts of love. The world's greatest writers, dramatists and composers have deeply profound love in its magical and poignant form, How can one forget

William Shakespeare's immortal classic "Romeo and Juliet," the touching movie and song-"Love is a Many Splendored Thing," and many other heart-rending stories.

Well, let us delightfully recall some meaningful sayings of LOVE as discerned by intuitive writers. Sir Walter Scott said, "Love is loveliest when embalmed in tears." Plato said, "Love is a grave mental disease." Leo Buscaglio-"Love isn't love unless given away." According to Franklin W. Bourdillon, "The light of a whole life dies when love is gone."

Pope John XXIII said, "He who has a heart full of love has always something to give." And Karl Menninger–– "Love cures people–– both ones who give it and the ones who receive it."

However, the best elucidation of love is the one that truly carries a spiritual connotation. Such as this one: "There is no greater love than this than to lay down his life for a friend." (Biblical scripture.) Above all, love each other deeply, because love covers a multitude of sins. (John 15:13, NLT) Psychologists comprehensively define love as "a complex, yet basically unified, as well as a feeling of empathy; the ability to enter into the feelings and experiences of one; pleasure in activity devoting thought, energy, time and all resources to the love one; and full of acceptance of the uniqueness and individuality of the one being loved."

Every righteous man in this world always seek and crave for real love for love is the essential energy that nurtures growth, the balm that brings healing when he is broken and succors him when he is downtrodden. When man receives the unconditional love of God, he begins to love himself and to love others.

Love will not save us from the pain of this life nor will

it protect us from the sorrow of death. However, love is the power of God within us that transcends pain and sorrow.

The power of love creates beautiful things to lift the spirit of the world. For the sake of love, we should be prepared to sacrifice in every way.

Let us recall the real qualities of a loving person. He is patient, kind, not envious, not proud, not rude, not self-seeking, not easily angered, keeps no record of wrongs, not happy with evil, and rejoices with the truth. These traits are the best passport to Heaven.

The Search for Meaning and Purpose in Life

"There is more to life than just
existing and have a pleasant time."
Friedrich von Schiller

One of the greatest existential psychoanalysts of all time is Victor Frankl. He is the exponent of "Logotherapy," a concept of a "will to meaning," that is, striving to see in life and fulfill a meaning and purpose. Today, people complain of a sense of meaninglessness and emptiness that Frankl termed as "existential frustration."

The Christian-oriented existentialist concluded that as long as man is still alive, even if he is in a state of helplessness or in an extremely deplorable situation, he should not lose hope for there is always a Divine Creator who can make things happen for him. One must fully accept and resign to whatever fate in this life for there is always a meaning and purpose that Almighty God has designed or plan for all of us in this world.

Today's people are becoming too materialistic and ambitious. They always desire to live-up with the

Joneses. They strive to luxuriously have a big house, a car or two, a colored television set, a personal computer, laptop, camera phones, a washing machine and other things that make life too comfortable. Yet, so many do not have the real meaning and purpose except for their own personal aggrandizement and pleasurable pursuit in life (self-centeredness).

Victor Frankl offers an interesting insight into this materialistic world that can help man understand how to live meaningfully. He says that "Life has meaning under all circumstances until we die. Generally, people have an innate will to meaning. This is our strongest motivation for living and action. Thus, the existential questions "Who am I?" "Where do I come from?" "Where am I going?" and "What is the purpose of my life?" are the guideposts to the real meaning of life.

According to Frankl's observation, "people have a lot to live on but very little to live for." For instance, most politicians have found their happiness through "under the table deals" (corruption); businessmen are happy robbing their customers and government through shady deals (i.e. smuggling) with huge profits; most people enjoy individualistic living *(kanya-kanya)* without showing concern *(paldalam)* for their poor *silingan* (neighbor), etc. Everybody is becoming a smart manipulator (a cheater) to succeed in life--definitely a satanic influence.

In order to truly fulfill the real meaning and purpose of this life, let us therefore be united in living as true Christians and ultimately loving and serving Almighty God through his people.

Quest of Simplicity

*"To be simple is to fix one's eye solely
on the simple truth of God at a
time when all 1 concepts are being
confused, distorted and turned upside
down. It is to be simple hearted."*
Dietrich Benhoeffer

Most spiritually-endowed people admire and understand the sterling virtue of simplicity for to them "simplicity is beauty." When I was a kid, I could not forget the Filipino leader, Soc Rodrigo, who spoke impressively on the subject of -"ONE." He said, "One is the simplest number and yet it signifies the greatest of meanings."

Apparently, many of our people today are caught in a web of rapid social and technological changes. Many Filipinos are striving hard and desire to live ambitiously in a much higher stratum of life-"keeping up with the Joneses." This is reflected in the expression-"want to be complete from A to Z (Not only for a multivitamin pill) but it means-if possible, to strive for health, beauty, and popularity. Nothing is wrong with these aims. However, the extremely stressful attempt to possess and accumulate wealth, power and prestige-through hell should bar the way"-is inevitably disastrous. Naturally, living always in a high gear like most of every ambitious type "A" personality certainly leads to an overload on one's health, then, bang!-sudden cardiovascular attack-the price to pay for a highly complicated pursuit in life.

Now let us focus and emulate the simple life philosophy of most great men who ever lived in this chaotic and too complexed world. They exemplified the winning beauty of simplicity in their thought, conduct and speech. They have a burning desire to simplify all that is complicated and to threat everything with the greatest naturalness and clarity.

Take for instance, Pope John XXIII (known as the pope who got a sense of humor). His life is driven by one grand simple idea: PEACE. Even in his words were so simple like a "parable." When the Jewish leaders visited him, he did not quote intricate doctrines to explain and overcome the century-old rift. He simply acted out like a man separated from his family. Pope John reached out to his visitors and simply said: "I am Joseph, your brother." (Genesis 45:4, NLT)

Simplicity was also exemplified by the great Hindu leader and pacifist Mahatma Gandhi, who focused his life with passion on his most lowly people when he called them, "the last, the least, the lowest, and the lost."

Another great man was Dr. Albert Scheitzer who had exceptionally shown his admiration for simplicity. The dedicated doctor spent the best years of his life serving the sick people in the jungle of Lamberene, Africa. His magnificent obsession: <u>Reverence for Life</u>. This is a true manifestation of great spirituality materialized. Why is Jesus so much loved by all in the world? Simple, because "<u>He went about doing good.</u>"

"The search for order and simplicity is a constant value in all religions," according to Martin E. Marty, the American writer.

The great lesson is clear: Let us simplify our life if we want to be optimally healthy, happier and live longer. We can do it. And why not?

The Healing Power of Vegetables

Our mothers were right in advising us to eat plenty of vegetables when we were still growing up. Too bad, we did not listen. We went on our way eating mostly fried foods, sweets, hamburgers and other junk foods until, unknowingly, we reached the "disease-prone age" and suffered the dire consequences of cancer, heart and kidney diseases, hypertension, obesity, diabetes and other stress related ailments, which took the lives of many relatively young people. Hence, this is a dismaying lesson for all. Let us therefore educate or children to eat more vegetables (and of course, fruits) to stave off the dreadful diseases to occur. Let us take the health benefits of some of our vegetables:

- **Carrots** are rich in alpha and beta-carotene, which prevent the development of cancers.
- **Celery** contains psoralens, which prevent psoriasis and lymphoma (cancer of the lymph nodes).
- **Cruciferous vegetables** such as broccoli, cauliflower, cabbage, lettuce, pechay, which contain sulfaraphane which boasts production of enzymes isothiocvnate that wash away chemical wastes. They also contain cancer-fighting carotenoids, anti-oxidants-lutein and zeaxanthin, which are very good for our eyes health; dithiothione, which promote glutathione that protects our body's cells (DNA).
- **Onions and garlic** contain alkyl sulfide, which rids the body in excreting carcinogenic chemicals. Garlic greatly helps in our metabolism and prevents the production of tumor cells.
- **Legumes** (beans, peas, etc.) are high in carbohydrates, fibers and good quality proteins and they are cholesterol-free. They are good

for diabetics for their insulin regulation, as well as prevent intestinal and colon cancers.

- **Mushrooms** contain selenium, which is good for immune function; prevent colon cancer as well as heart diseases.
- **Potatoes** contain catechols, which benefits immune function warding off infection and other diseases.

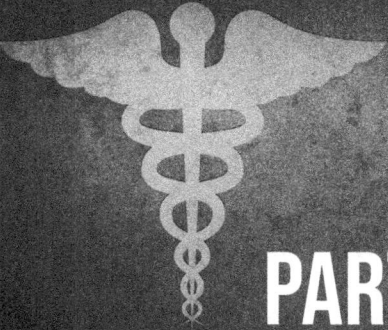

PART II

BODILY DISORDERS THAT SLOW US DOWN

Causes of Fatigue

> *"Slow down and keep the even rhythm*
> *of God, the source of all energy."*
>   Anonymous

Normally in life, one experiences being fatigued due to an overexertion or physical work. However, there are some people who gets tired easily for some unknown reason. Let us then unravel some factors causing weakness or loss of essential energy in man and prevent them to happen.

Doctors claim that about one often people (many of them women) maybe troubled by daytime fatigue due to physical or mental exhaustion. Possibly, the common cause may stem from some factors such as sleep problems, the first symptom of an approaching illness or any medical conditions, side-effects of medications, or something as simple as not drinking enough water. More often, probably, the likely cause may be lack of exercise, an unbalanced diet, stress, smoking, alcohol drinking and simply not getting enough rest.

In a busy life, let us take for instance some common causes of debility. Undoubtedly, some individuals are simply overloaded with too many responsibilities that make them feel so weak or tired. From early morning to late in the evening, they saddle themselves up by tedious works from the office the whole day and when they arrive home in the late afternoon. They hurry to go marketing and upon arriving home, they still cook for supper and still they do all the household chores (good for those families who have reliable helpers, like helpful husbands, grown-up children and relatives to assist). Worse still, the overworked wife may still have to serve an unreasonably strict and overdemanding husband in bed.

Aside from the hectic physical activities I mentioned, there are still other factors that bring about weakness in man, such as:

- Stressful emotional or psychological disorders–– shocking news, suffering from excruciating pain, confronted with a frightening object, etc., depression, anxiety, sapping the person's energy.
- Sick with a serious, medical or neurological illness like congestive heart failure, uncontrollable diarrhea causing electrolyte imbalance, shock, hepatitis, fainting spell, market loss of blood, cancer, emphysema, etc.
- Severe infections caused by virulent bacteria and viral agents (i.e. colds, influenza, pneumonia, tuberculosis, dengue, etc.).
- Intake of toxic substances (i.e. drugs, alcohol, poisons like lead or mercury).

- Eating of unbalanced diet with faulty nutritional values (i.e. too much saturated fats, too salty and too much sugar, lack of vitamins and minerals like iron causing severe anemia, obesity, diabetes, mellitus, etc.). All these conditions result in weakness

An advice from Julio Silverio--"Avoid the gray sickness, half awake, half asleep, half alive and half dead." Hence, definitely fatigue is one of man's greatest enemies. Therefore, we have to prevent it by finding ways to cope with stress and overworked as well by consulting our medical specialist before fatigue may load to undue physical or mental symptoms as anxiety, depression and untimely death.

Alzheimer's Disease (A.D.)

*"Alzheimer's Disease is a single most
significant health and social crisis
of the 21st century. It is predicted
to reach 65 million sufferers
worldwide in the year 2030."*
World Statistics

A close family friend of ours had to give up a very lucrative job in Manila. She came home to Negros just to fully attend to her elderly (70-year old) mother who was diagnosed of having Alzheimer's Disease.

Let us learn the facts of this "modem" scourge of the century. This disorder was discovered by a German neurologist, Dr. Alois Alzheimer. This disease was formerly identified with dementia (general impairment of the brain in the elderly). In AD, there is a steady deterioration of brain function resulting in continuous loss of memory, the inability to recognize friends and even family members, and of personality and mental deterioration. It can start as early as the age of 40 but it is prevalent in the aged. AD is said to account for half of all serious mental impairments of persons over the age of 65.

The consistent pathological feature shows an atrophy (shrinkage) of the cerebral cortex (outer layer of the brain) which is mostly concerned with intellectual and social functioning. The micro or histopathological findings consistently show tangles or whorls of fibers within the nerve cells and deposits of amyloid (a semisolid protein complex as seen in many degenerative diseases). These abnormal changes are scattered throughout the cortex.

Authorities claim that AD could possibly be due to viruses; lack of enzyme choline-acetyl transferase; high levels of aluminum or mercury in the brain. Heredity plays a role. Scientists role out stress as a probable factor. Smoking is a high risk for it causes abulia (loss of initiative or will power).

Symptoms vary considerably. Prominent symptoms include: forgetfulness-especially recollection of recent events. Example: forgetting his name; losing his way home from office; forgetting to tum off the oven; misplaces articles or asks repeated questions already answered; etc. The extreme memory loss could interfere with normal work and social networking. As the disease progresses, the victim of AD becomes confused, frustrated and extremely irritable. As the condition advances, the patient becomes extremely restless, and must be watched so that he/she does not wander away or is placed in a dangerous situation. Many AD patients do endless repetitions of meaningless actions.

At the moment, medical science does not still know how to prevent or treat AD. However, exponential medical consultants can help the patient and family handle the many problems with the use of medications when they arise. Otherwise, hospitalization is a must.

General management and prevention of AD:

- Advice patient to continue daily routine-exercise as usual; keep in touch with friends, etc.
- Provide a round-the-clock health care.
- Eat foods rich in vitamins B6 and 12, vitamin E, and folic acid. Eat whole grains, soy-based products or low fat dairy products, lentils and leafy greens. Eat at least one piece of fish every week to improve cognitive functioning as suggested by studies.
- Develop mental fitness-Example: Lifelong mental exercises (solving crossword puzzles, reading, card games, etc.).
- Avoid toxic materials–– i.e. mercury or silver tooth fillings; smoking; polluted water, etc.

AGING-The Seasoning of Life

*"To look old is much better
than to be dead."*

Anonymous

Acceptably, aging is a very normal phenomenon in life that happens between birth and death. It has four major stages--childhood, adolescence, adulthood, and senescense. Let us focus on the last stage-"old age" which concerns most health-conscious people.

Majority of our people have a negative attitude towards getting old. A long time ago in the history of civilization old age or known as the "Golden Age" is equated with wisdom, power, and great experience. These great elderly men like the Greek figures–– Aristotle, Plato, Homer, etc.; great statesmen and heroes-Julius Caesar, Churchill, MacArthur; writers as Shakespeare, Dickens, Hemingway; our Laurel, Recto and many other brilliant elderly men (past 60's).

Today, many are dismayed and many dislike old age for it is associated with decline, deterioration, weakness and death. Nobody wants to die young. If someone compliments you-"you have not changed, you still look much younger than your age!" Then you feel good. But we cannot escape from the natural ravages of aging such as the wrinkling of the skin. Weakening of one's strength, graying of hair, aching of joints, failing of vision, cardiovascular problems, etc. A certain H. Fritch says, "Age is quality of the mind. If you have left your dreams behind; if hope is cold; if you no longer look ahead; if your ambition's fire is dead; then you are old." Someone also said that, "Being over seventy years old is like being engaged in a war. All our friends are going or gone and we survive among the dead and dying as on a battlefield."

Today, in the advent of advanced health discoveries countless of lives have been saved and millions of people have prolonged their life span. In Japan alone, there are people who are living beyond 100 years mark. In Pakistan, a report says that there is a "Village of Centarians" where senior citizens thrived. Consistent factors in achieving a much long life in these agricultural areas are: Simple diet of vegetables, fruits, fish or farm animals like goats, fouls; physically active lifestyle; less stress, and a strong family and community solidarity.

The multimillion cosmetic industry and plastic surgery business have contributed to the physical outlook of the moneyed middle aged and some elderly. For instance, a "face-lift" can transform one's nose, lips, wrinkled skin, etc. to look beautiful and youthful. Plastic surgeons can now improve any ugly part of the body by cutting or even adding some tissues of the body to make it appear younger.

The secret of achieving healthy and much longer life span are:

- Always be a good and loving person.
- Avoid vices and bad habits.
- Be active and have a regular aerobic exercise.
- Have a regular medical, dental, and visual check-up.
- Be moderate in all your activities.
- Have a strong Faith and develop a good Spiritual Life.

Essential Factors to be observed in Aging Process

Inevitably, man grows older every minute in a day without knowing it. He only realizes that aging is beginning to creep in his mind and body because his memory is no longer sharp; he misses to name his children, respectably. In doing his physical activities, he feels some aches and pains in his body, so much so that he begins to be extra careful in his movements and doing his daily routines.

Authorities suggests some useful activities that

would help minimize the pangs of growing old. Here are some suggestions:

1. Observe proper diet, exercise, and get enough rest and sleep.
2. Continue doing your wholesome activities in life.
3. Do things in moderation,
4. Refrain from vices and bad habits like smoking, drinking and drug abuse.
5. Don't let your emotions rule you--like useless anxiety, anger and heated arguments.
6. Seek early medical assistance from proper authorities for any health problem.
7. Cultivate a prayerful and a strong spiritual life.

Supplements that Slow Down Aging

"Growing old is not bad when you consider the alternative."
Maurice Chevalier

As man ages his body begins to slow the production of enzymes, hormones and other nutrients which are needed to feel young and to look young. Experts say that we can add years to our lives by replacing these nutrients with supplements.

Here are the newer vital top-selling supplements sold in drug stores and groceries in our markets:

- **COENZYME Q10.** This enzyme regulates electrical currents in the energy producing mitochondria of our cells. Co Q10 strengthens the heart, prevents and treats cancer like breast cancer, fast recovery from illness or surgery, fights gum disease and it may help muscular dystrophy.

Dose: A daily dose of 30 to 50 mg will suffice. Some may take up to 100 to 300 mg a day, if your doctor approves.

- **DHEA** (Dehydro-Epiano-Adrosterone). This is a natural steroid hormone which declines as we age. This improves immune function, memory, low energy, lupus, depression and post-menopausal sex drive. It also protects against heart attack and various cancers.

  Dose: One 50 mg tab, daily for men and 25 mg tab, daily for women.

- **MELATONIN.** A hormone secreted by the pineal gland in the brain. Infants produce a large amount of melatonin. But as the person ages the pineal body calcifies, causing the elderly to suffer from **insomnia** meaning the inability to sleep. Melatonin delays aging. It is now used to prevent **jet lag.**

  Dose: Take 3 to 5 mg melatonin at bedtime for those who have difficulty in sleeping.

- **VALERIAN ROOT** (natural vitamin). One of the relaxing herbs. It enables one to relax both physically and mentally when one is overworked, tensed and under stressed.

Dose: Take 1 to 2 mg valerian capsule before bedtime.

- **GINGKO BILOBA.** This herb enhances memory, improves mental capability and memory loss when aging, and delays onset of dementia in old age as well as Alzheimer's disease.

   Dose: Take 100 to 240 mg. two times a day, or three times a day.

These supplements are the most important ones.

The Anti-Aging Benefits of Vitamin E

A lot of people actually are unaware of the anti-aging properties and other benefits of Vitamin E. They only know from studies that Vitamin E is only good for human sexual development such as fertility and anti-abortion properties. But scientific studies have revealed more benefits of this wonderful vitamin.

Vitamin E is a natural antioxidant, a fatty acid found in vegetable oils. It is also known for its healing properties and its ability to give the immune system a significant boost.

Anti-aging researchers have called Vitamin E the most crucial vitamin supplement to ward off the disease of aging. Indeed, many top experts and researchers personally take Vitamin E for this reason.

Researchers have discovered that Vitamin E lengthens life as proven by a number of studies. Other significant findings of Vitamin E are: it fights heart attacks and strokes. In fact, the American Heart Association has declared that Vitamin E is one of the most important supplements one can take to keep his heart healthy. Studies at Tufts University showed that older people derived substantial immunity benefits from taking Vitamin E supplement and that the vitamin was also well tolerated. The remarkable immune system benefits came from taking Vitamin E supplements ranging from 400/U to 800/U per day.

Another benefit is Vitamin E prevents cataract formation. Cataract can lead to blindness, if not removed earlier surgically.

Vitamin E can also fight cancer. Those taking Vitamin E supplement, a major study in Finland had claimed that it could prevent less vulnerable to cancer.

Vitamin E has been shown to be effective against arthritis inflammation and helps ease morning stiffness.

Food sources of Vitamin E: It is found in fatty foods as nuts and seeds, whole grains, wheat germ and vegetable oils such as sunflower, soybean and corn. One cannot get enough Vitamin E in food alone. So he must take vitamin supplement to obtain maximum anti-aging action.

Caution: Toxic level at dose above 3,800/U daily. Signs of Toxicity: High blood pressure, diarrhea, stomach upset.

Anorexia Nervosa

*"I am not going to starve just
so I can live a little longer."*
Irene Peter

When the famous international singer, Karen Carpenter, suffered and died of Anorexia Nervosa, the whole world was puzzled and questioned why the young and talented singer had to succumb to the particular malady. Many other young girls who belonged to the upper-middle class family also died due to this impaired weight-related illness-the morbid fear of becoming fat. The impact of the most prevailing belief among the present-day teenagers and young women which had greatly influenced by the mass media (i.e. Beauty magazines depicting fashionable models, etc.) in promoting the idea that the only approved and acceptable "body beautiful" in society is the slim (thin) willowy look, but extremely hated the fat (overweight) figure which looks so horrible to them.

Now let us unravel the abnormality of this disease. "Anorexia" means "without appetite" and "nervosa" means "nervous in origin." This is a serious and deadly type of an eating disorder common among young women characterized by self-starvation leading to extreme weight loss to the point of malnutrition and starvation.

Statistics report that about 95% of anorexics are female, most are teenagers and young women corning from the upper middle class families. About one (1) in 200 women of this age and social class I estimated to suffer from anorexia nervosa.

The characteristic features include a distorted body-image, and extreme fear of obesity, refusal to maintain a minimal normal body weight, and absence of menstrual periods. This particular illness could be fatal because an anorexia can literally starve to death while she continues to think mistakenly as "fat" and need to diet. The result is not only an unattractively skinny appearance, but also an end to menstrual periods, a subtle reminder of the happier days of childhood.

Psychologically speaking, anorexics are said to be

suffering from an unconscious deep-seated conflicts. Although they seem to appear "normal" or "perfect" and compliant to the wishes of all. Anorexics are said to be scared that in her childhood, she might become fat and develop large pendulous breasts, big bulging hips and abdomen and too large thighs, hence, they obsessively observe a strict diet regimen. They really have a distorted concept of body-image. Hence, they induce themselves not to eat, or force to vomit, use laxatives, or overly engage in vigorous exercise just so to maintain a very thin look.

Treatment involves hospitalization to encourage the subject to gain weight. Some anorexic patients become too thin or emaciated. Management is done through behavior modification and intensive psychotherapy as well as medical intervention to save the patient from deep depression, starvation, malnourishment and death. Hence this needs a team approach by a medical internist, psychiatrist and dietitian (nutritionist). Therapy must also include the cooperation of the family members. Early management is needed once a doctor makes a diagnosis of anorexia nervosa. Treatment is quite difficult especially when it is already in the advance stage. It had been reported that about 10-20% of anorexic patients die.

So, young girls beware of too much slim fests. Just maintain an average healthy-looking body but control your too much eating of ice cream, fats, sweets, and potato chips. Okay?

CANCER-The Dreaded Modern scourge

"Cancer are rebellious cells in a community of law-abiding cells."
Medical Report

Cancer today is considered a modem deadly disease, although it is not unknown in ancient times. The Greek has called cancer as a "crab" probably because of its clawing crab-like growth. The incident of cancer has been increasing dramatically in years, primarily due to a number of known and undetermined factors that harm the body such as irritants as tobacco in smoke. Air pollutants in vehicles, factories, farms additives in foods, viral and bacterial infections, stressful habits, and abusive lifestyles causing "psychosomatic" illnesses, etc.

Based on reliable statistics, cancer is second only to heart disease. And if the present trends continue, cancer may well overtake heart disease as the number 1 cause of death.

Let us review the early signs of cancer growth. (UN Studies)

1. A sore (lesion) of the body that does not heal.
2. Unusual bleeding or discharge.
3. A nagging cough or hoarseness.
4. Thickening or lump in the breast or elsewhere.
5. Change in bowel and/or bladder habits.
6. Indigestion or difficulty in swallowing.
7. Obvious change in wart or mole.

Do not delay if you suspect an unusual growth or changes in your body. Please refer immediately to your doctor. Cancer prevention starts in our plate.

Researchers have discovered foods that possess potential anti-cancer properties. These foods should be a part of our all-around healthy diet which helps lower the risk of cancer formation in our body. For instance:

- Eating less meat and less high fat, cutting down the amount of cooking fats and oils can minimize the risk of colon, breast, prostate and other cancers.

- Minimize the eating of salt-cured and smoked foods such as bacon, ham, smoked sausages, and too charred or burnt barbecues of pork which are believed to be carcinogenic.
- Eat diet high in whole grains, cereals, fruits, vegetables, and other sources of fibers for they help reduce the risk for colon cancer.
- Eat more fruits rich in anti-oxidants and vitamin C (citrus fruits, guavas, guyabanos, pineapple), and vitamin A (carrots, squash, and other yellow fruits), and more vegetables (cabbage, broccoli, cauliflower, kale, Brussels sprouts) and legumes (beans, garbanzos, etc.) plus foods rich in lycopene (tomatoes, melons) which prevent prostate cancer.
- Include Kelp or "sea vegetables" (Lato, guso-- seaweeds) plus the colorful berries (black and blue berries, strawberry and grape seeds), sunflower seeds and nuts (almond, walnut), oils (olive oil, canola oil), green tea and healthy seasoning–– garlic, onions, mustard, ginger.

When you go to the market to buy some groceries, be sure to include the above foods that have anti-cancer properties. Go fit and healthy!

Baldness

*"Baldness is said to be a crisis
coming to a head."*

Anonymous

God must have a good purpose in adoring man with hair in his head to enhance his looks. For protection, to signify strength, fort sexual attraction, to reflect on his age and character, etc.

Hair has significant meanings. The Holy Bible explicitly showed the power of unusual strength on Samson's hair. But when Delilah cut his hair when he was deadly drunk. Samson lost all his strength. We term the process in Psychiatry as **Castration.** Any person who loses his power to defend himself is said to be suffering from **Castration Complex.** However, the famous Hollywood actor, Yul Bryner who sported a shaven head, appeared to be too masculine in his looks, while Shaolin Monks and Cadets with short hair appeared normal, clean and physically fit.

Baldness (alopecia) is the partial or complete loss of hair on the head. This may be caused by hereditary tendency, aging, infection, certain drugs, radiation, injury or disease (tumor), hormonal (lack of androgen) may contribute to it. Baldness can begin as early as 15 or 16 years old. It is rare in women occurring during the menopausal age and usually involves only the thinning of the hair around the crown area, believed to be due to hormonal cause.

Temporary baldness occurs sometimes-up to 3 or 4 months following a severe illness; a lowered pituitary or thyroid activity, pregnancy, early syphilis, birth-control pills. **Crash** dieting or malnutrition, or certain medication, or too much Vitamin A. When the cause is no longer present, the missing hair usually returns.

There is a rare kind of baldness called **spotty baldness.** The cause is unknown. This is termed as **Alopecia Areata.** It affects the head and beard. If it occurs in adulthood, the prognosis is good. But when it begins in childhood, the outcome is unfavorable.

Permanent baldness results when the scalp is scarred by burns, other injuries or serious diseases like severe bacterial infections, severe ringworm of the scalp, lupus erethematosus and certain slow growing tumors.

There is no satisfactory treatment at this time to cure or prevent baldness. Although, there are already now **hair management** like **hair transplant** and the **use of hair lotion** to promote the growth of hair follicles. The **use of wigs** can be tried, too.

Don't Ignore HEADACHES

"A headache resembles a Crown of Thorns worn by persons obsessed with negative conscience."

Anonymous

One of the most common health complaints of people is headache. There are several types of headaches depending on their causes. Significantly, one should not ignore a headache for it may become an ominous start of a very serious condition like a brain tumor or cancerous growth.

Medical authorities claim that majority or more than 90% of headaches are caused by tension. There are four major types of headaches; 1. Tension Headache; 2. Vascular Headache like migraine; 3. Inflammation Headache like Sinusitis; 4. Traction Headache due to tumor or cancer. Let me discuss the first two (2) types of Headaches.

Tension Headache is the most common type of headache. This usually occurs during times of emotional and physical turmoil or stress. The pain is usually felt in the muscles all over the head radiating to the jaw, the neck, back and shoulders. It could be felt as a pressure or feeling like a tight band around one's head or severe pain like a vise grip. Some sufferers feel like a dull pressing, burning sensation above the eyes. One can rarely pinpoint the source of the pain. There is no specific personality type associated with tension headache. But it is commonly related to chronic or long-standing tension and anxiety. Unresolved stress can aggravate tension headache. Hence, it is the most recurrent kind of headache that afflicts the young and adult patients who are easily tense or nervous.

Migraine Headache is a severe type of headache that is usually one-sided, accompanied with visual disturbances (extreme sensitiveness to light, etc.) and a throbbing or piercing type of pain. Victims experience an "aura" like light flashing, etc. before the attack. Persons prone to suffer migraine are the Obsessive-Compulsive Personality. They are perfectionists, excessively orderly, and success-oriented. Emotionalism can trigger migraine attacks.

PREVENTION AND TREATMENT:

- Keep a diary of headache symptoms to keep track of what event, food or substance causes your headache.
- At the first sign of headache, try to go to a quiet and dark place and relax. Sleeping can relieve migraine.
- Apply a cold pack or cloth on your forehead or painful area. Heat makes migraine worse.
- Learn a progressive relaxation exercise.

- You may take a safe pain-reliever like paracetamol or ibuprofen.
- Some herbal preparations like "honey and cinnamon" can relieve pain.
- If headache persists consult your doctor who can physically examine you with the aid of needed Laboratory procedures the exact cause of your headache. He can also judiciously prescribe a good and safe pain-reliever.

Dizziness and Vertigo

The above serious symptoms of dizziness commonly occur to young Filipino patients especially to children who utterly lack iron in their diet because they dislike vegetables, and they also suffer parasitism that contribute to deprivation of iron in the blood.

Many School Physicians have been observing and treating children who are suffering from severe anemia-a disease or illness characterized by recurrent dizziness, light headedness, weakness, pallor, poor memory, faintness, and at times nausea and vomiting. Anemia with constant dizziness is a major cause of poor scholastic performance and failure in school. But simple dizziness can easily be treated with proper diet and taking palatable iron preparation and other vitamin supplements.

Vertigo, on the other hand is more serious and an alarming nervous disturbance which needs immediate attention and treatment. Neurologists define vertigo as the loss of the sense of balance, equilibrium and position. The patient complains that the room seems to be spinning or that the whole world seems to be whirling around. Vertigo is accompanied with nausea, vomiting, total weakness and a faint feeling, aside from staggering and falling down helplessly. The patient is forced to close his eyes to minimize the unpleasant sensation.

The most common causes of Vertigo are:

1. Disturbance in the inner ear (cochlea) where the sense of balance is controlled.
2. Ear infection involving the middle and inner ear.
3. Blockage of the Eustachian Tube.
4. Excessive use of alcohol and tobacco.
5. Abrupt change of body position, getting up from lying-down position.
6. Sudden spasm of blood vessels in the brain.
7. Hemorrhage of the brain (stroke).
8. Encephalitis or meningitis of the brain.
9. Otosclerosis of the hearing apparatus.
10. Brain tumor, etc.

Treatment: See a Neurologist immediately!

PAIN: Human Equalizer

*"Adversity reveals genius,
prosperity conceals."*

Horace

From birth to the last breath, in one way or another, man experiences pain and suffering in various ways. No human being is ever spared from the reality of the existence of pain. In this philosophical sense, pain is said to be a great human equalizer and proving the very fact that all men are truly created equal. As a doctor, I may be able to describe or define pain in its physiological context. Medically speaking, pain is said to be an unpleasant or uncomfortable sensation that ranges from mild irritation to excruciating agony. Pain is the most common reported symptom felt by anyone as a result of a disease or disorder.

Man by nature desires to live in a state of good health at any cost and avoids suffering of pain of any kind. This wish is unrealistic and a sort of a denial (defense mechanism) for life without pain is not life. God never promises to take away pain but He allows it to happen. Theologians say that pain purifies, tempers, humiliates and makes man more compassionate towards his neighbors and it could make him a better person. Pain is part of our deliverance. God promised His Eternal Kingdom to those who could face and endure the pains and sufferings of this life. This is a great lesson of "No cross, no crown" philosophy.

Let us be reminded of the major sources of psychic (emotional) pain in life which include the extreme deprivations of biological, psychological, social and spiritual needs of man.

Let me cite some examples:

- Biological causes include: intractable insomnia, exhaustion or overfatigue (i.e. Burnt-out Syndrome); extreme hunger and starvation; addiction; brain damage due to drugs and alcohol; lack of exercise; effects of severe infections; cancer, etc.
- Psychological causes include: sudden loss of loved ones through death or separation; impoverishment; utter lack of love and affection (cruelties); meaninglessness; powerlessness; bankruptcy; burned alive; trapped; crippling

accidents; disfigurement; war; famine; epidemics; traumatic catastrophies or tragedies, etc.

- <u>Social causes</u>: impaired interpersonal relationships; abandonment; constant quarrels; living in a terror-stricken area; bad and hostile neighbors; ostracism; absence of friends; divorce; infidelity; etc.

- <u>Spiritual causes</u>: atheism; agnosticism; hedonism; materialism; severe immortality of state of sinfulness; a godless life; demon-possessed; superstitious living; witchcraft (voodoo), etc.

Sleep Disorder

*"Sleep grants us oblivion
from our daily worries."*

Anonymous

One of the paramount aims of this column is not only to inform and educate, but to correct misconceptions. Many of our people are seeking the help of their doctors because they believe that insomnia is a disease. No, it is not a disease but it is a symptom of a disease-a sleep disorder. Generally, most if not all, mental and emotional disorders usually start to show itself, first with the symptom of sleeplessness or what is commonly called as, **Insomnia.**

Insomnia is defined as the inability to sleep during normal sleeping hours when there is no reason for wakefulness.

Statistics show that one-third of all adults cannot get a good sleep at one time or another. As people get older they are prone to have insomnia. Once one turns 40, you are 40% more likely to experience some degree of insomnia. Hence, as people get older, they tend to sleep less.

What are the possible causes of insomnia? The condition is often associated with emotional or psychological problems, and also physical disorders, as well as conditions in the immediate environment. It often occurs with such emotional disturbances such as fear, anxiety, depression and nervousness. Among physical disorders that lead to insomnia are urination problems, heart trouble high blood pressure, infections of the ear, tooth causing aches, etc., back pains, allergies, stomach cramps, diarrhea, constipation, and others.

Less serious causes of insomnia can be caused by environmental conditions such as bright lights, noise, cold or very warm bedroom, lack of ventilation, too many or few bedclothes, pests like mosquitoes, bugs, squeaky beds, uncomfortable beds, hunger pangs, too much coffee, tea, strong chocolate, cola drinks, other beverages containing stimulants and some medications. Paradoxically, some drugs to promote sleep can cause insomnia. Too much siesta can also cause insomnia.

Some ways of preventing or coping with simple insomnia include:

    a. Taking a 10 or 15 minute walk before bedtime.
    b. Taking a warm bath.
    c. Drinking warm milk (milk contains **tryptophan,** a substance that naturally promotes drowsiness).
    d. Reading a "boring" book or watching a "dull" TV show.
    e. Don't eat and drink heavily before retiring. Indigestion and a full stomach won't

bring about sleep. Besides, you may suffer *"bangungot"* (hemorrhagic pancreatitis or a heart attack).

f. Picture a tranquil scene-beautiful meadow, serene lake, etc. Focus thoughts on peace, harmony, happiness, etc.

g. Don't bring nagging problems in bed.

h. Never forget to sincerely pray. Who knows it might be your last night. As a clergy says, "You may rest in peace!" (Meaning, make your night very peaceful indeed, my friend.)

Warning: Taking a sleeping pill should be discussed with your doctor. Anti-insomnia pills (hypnotic) are definitely habit-forming and to be taken only for "intractable insomnia," and to be carefully supervised by an experienced doctor. OK?

Nondrug Treatment for Insomnia:

1. Go to bed only when you are sleepy.
2. Put off the light immediately when going to bed.
3. Do not read or watch television in bed since these are activities that you do when awake.
4. If you are not asleep within 20 minutes get out of bed and sit and relax in another room until you are sleepy tired again. Relaxation can include tensing and relaxing one's muscles or using visual imagery which involves closing one's eyes and concentrating on some calm or pleasant image for several minutes.
5. Repeat step 4 as often as required and also if you are awake for any long periods of time.

6. Set the alarm to the same time each morning so that your time in waking is the same. Avoid oversleeping as a primary cause of insomnia the next night.
7. Do not nap during the day because it will throw you off your sleep schedule that night.
8. Follow this program rigidly for several weeks to establish an efficient and regular pattern of sleep.

However, if these cognitive behavioral techniques don't work, it indicates that you are suffering from deep seated unresolved conflicts in your life. You are therefore advised to see a Psychiatrist to resolve your **unconscious problems** to be able to fully enjoy all your insomnia-free night.

Hyperventilation-a risky acting-out syndrome

Medical reports claim that many patients who died with hyperventilation syndrome were misdiagnosed as "heart attack." So, we have to know the causes as well as the symptoms of these clinical entities. Hyperventilation syndrome is medically described as a condition that occurs when a person breathes very rapidly and deeply that causes the carbon dioxide (CO_2) in his blood to a very low level affecting the normal CO_2-O_2 balance of the body, thus causing the common symptom of Hyperventilation: Shortness of breath; Fast breathing; Chest pain stimulating a heart attack; Weakness and dizziness; Numbness and tingling sensation around the mouth, hands and feet; Pounding and racing heartbeat; Feeling that you can't get enough air; Light headedness;

Feeling like you might pass out or faint. If the attack is severe, you might lose your consciousness.

Causes:

Studies have shown that hyperventilation is common in anxiety disorder. Severe stress could also trigger it. But the most vulnerable ones are the hysterical personalities "Cleopatra Complex," example the actresses who feigned or acted out their feelings because their desires were not met. For instance, a fearful mother witnessing her two sons seriously fighting held her chest and deeply breathing fast. And suddenly she fell down on the floor, gasping and panting as if she was having a "heart attack." The sight of the mother on the floor stopped the furious fight of the two sons.

Management:

- Rebreathing Bag-Get a clean paper bag and let the patient have his nose and mouth in the bag and take one breath every 10 seconds, inhaling and exhaling without stopping until the level of CO_2 is normally stabilized. Do this for about 5 to 15 minutes until symptoms gradually disappear.
- The patient should be advised to see his counselor to prevent recurrence of his unresolved conflicts and attack of hyperventilation.

The Essence of Rest and Sleep

"Sleep is the best cure for
walking troubles."

Cervantes

Psychologists recognize that rest and sleep are one of the most essential biological needs of man like food. Rest and sleep are mostly needed in the building or restoration process ("the wear") of the loss of cells and other bodily tissues ("the tear") during the waking active activities of man. If man will be deprived of sleep, an unpleasant condition is created known in psychiatry as Insomnia (see Sleep Disorder write-up above).

Speaking of rest, one of the most valuable times to take a daytime rest is after a few minutes after lunch when blood is shunted from the brain to the actively working digestive system. The brief noon rest is known as "cat-nap." Many world famous leaders like Winston Churchill of England found that taking a 10 to 30-minute nap during noontime daily increases stamina, concentration and lifespan. This short restful process will refresh one's feelings as well as revitalizes a person's activities the rest of the day. One does not have to sleep necessarily for several hours in the afternoon.

Duration of sleep varies largely. The average hours of sleep recommended for adults is 6 to 8 hours of uninterrupted sleep at night. Pope Leo XIII needed only 3 hours of sleep but others like former US President Woodrow Wilson and many others used to sleep for 9 hours a night. Babies need much more hours of sleep for growth and development. But adults and old people need much less hours of sleep. A nap at noon (about 30 minutes) is also good for most workers.

Let me close by saying that a sound sleep is very

vital to our body needs and health for it enables us to feel rested, invigorated and alive. Sleep is considered to be nature's sweet restorer. It allows man to temporarily escape from the world's problems. Sometimes sleep gives us a glimpse of a fleeting pleasure that we enjoy in a beautiful dream as well as a taste of hell in a terrifying nightmare.

Panic Attack

Some women experience panic attacks despite the fact that they happen to appear externally unruffled and "normal." For instance, a high-level woman executive of a corporation became constantly afraid that she might have an attack (panic) in front of her staff. In fact, she got anxious often that she finally lost her job. However, she submitted herself for psychiatric management and was successfully treated. She transferred to another less stressful work and became a healthy, happy, and capable worker.

Panic disorder is characterized by recurrent overwhelming anxiety attacks and nervousness. The attacks are characterized by a sudden onset of intense apprehension, fearfulness, or terror, often associated with feelings of impending doom.

The predisposing factor occurs in situations where separation anxiety frequently takes place. This is the common anxiety experienced in childhood when the overprotected child develops a strong attachment with the mother. When the mother leaves, the overprotected child becomes anxious, cries, and feels helpless.

Usually, the symptoms of panic disorder are similar to that of fear, yet the victim does not employ a defense mechanism to manage or control the attack. The most common symptoms experienced by the individuals are dyspnea (difficulty of breathing), palpitation (rapid heartbeat), chest pain or discomfort, choking or smothering sensation, dizziness, vertigo, unsteady feelings, feeling of unreality, paresthesia (numbness), hot and cold flashes, sweating, trembling or shaking, and fear of dying, going crazy, or doing something uncontrollable during an attack.

Treatment:

Seek psychiatric help (i.e. short-term supportive psychotherapy). Reassurance and support, not only verbal, but attitudinal as well. Environmental modification-take away victim from stressful situations; change detrimental lifestyles. Behavioral modification by applying deconditioning process. Family Therapy. Medications-the use of a minor tranquilizer to control rattled nerves; may also use antidepressant if depressive symptoms occur.

Parkinson's Disease

> *"We classify disease as error, which nothing but truth or mind can heal."*
> Mary Baker Eddy

Parkinson is a relatively common disease that affects generally the elderly. The late Pope Paul II suffered from it. A number of Filipinos are victimized by this neurological disorder.

Parkinson's disease is believed to be caused by a chemical imbalance in the brain-as shown by a low level of a neurotransmitter called dopamine-a chemical used in transmitting nerve impulses and responsible for rapid smooth movements of the limbs.

The classical symptoms are: tremors (shaking), especially of the hands and fingers at rest; stiffness of the limbs as shown by the "cogwheel rigidity" (occurring when the arm is pulled straight from a flexed position, the arm moves in a jerky fashion as if controlled by a ratchet like that is found in a cogwheel); there is difficulty initiating and the slowing of movements; a masklike face; walking (gait) disturbance (e.g. the person has trouble stopping an action once it has been initiated); and dementia ensues as shown by memory loss. About 50% of patients with Parkinson's disease suffer from depression; other symptoms include decreased blinking, a stooped posture and increased salivation (drooling of saliva).

Treatment modalities:

- Doctor prescribes levodopa to help the brain manufacture more of its own dopamine, coupled with drugs known as anticholinergics to reduce tremors, rigidity and drooling––(e.g. Bromocriptine).
- Help the patient function normally as possible. A program of regular exercise (physical therapy); the use of wheel chair or walking, a nutritious diet rich in high fiber foods to combat constipation and other needed B-complex vitamins and other deficiencies.
- May join a support group, if there are any, or encourage the help of family and friends for emotional support, and most importantly is to prepare his spiritual health (soul) for the inevitable Final Exit from this sinful world.

MENOPAUSE-The Female "Midlife Crisis"

Why is it that there are women who are seriously affected and suffer utter confusion during this particular period of life and there are those women who are not at all bothered by it? Let us find out why is this so.

Menopause is the normal, natural stage in a woman's life when her menstruation and ovulation cycles stop, ending her reproductive years. Also called climacteric or the change of life, it occurs around age 50 but can start anywhere between the ages of 40 to 60. During the years immediately preceding its onset, menstrual periods may become scant and irregular.

Scientists do not fully understand what causes menopause but they believe that it is triggered when the female sex glands, the ovaries, stop responding to the gonadotropic (sex gland) hormones that are secreted by the pituitary gland to control normal function of the ovaries. The ovaries' subsequent decline in the production of the female hormone estrogen sets off the bodily changes.

The physical symptoms of menopause include the following:

- Hot flashes (a warm and flushed feeling that comes over the face, neck, and chest and lasts a few minutes at a time but recurs throughout the day).
- Excessive perspiring, dryness in the vagina (which can lead to painful or difficult intercourse).
- Pounding heartbeat or palpitation, joint pains, headaches, itching skin, increased facial hair, and decreased armpit or pubic hair.

The nonphysical or psychological symptoms are the following:

- Depression
- Anxiety
- Irritability
- Apprehension
- Decrease ability to concentrate
- Lack of confidence
- Insomnia

For the management of the physical symptoms, please consult your Ob-Gyn specialist. And for the nonphysical or psychological symptoms, see a Psychiatrist.

What to do with "Midlife Crisis" in Men

One of the inevitable disturbing events in life that every man should prepare and defend himself with is "Midlife Crisis." To a woman, this is commonly called "Menopause".

Midlife Crisis has been affecting adversely countless of men throughout the world since time immemorial. Midlife or "prime of life" is a phrase used by the Greeks more than two thousand years ago. This is the very time of life (about 50) as the ideal age when one is most balanced between the age of youth and old age referred to as the "golden mean" of life.

However, midlife crisis affects men at different times. It can start during one's mid-thirties, late forties, and onwards (delayed). Midlife Crisis is often referred to as the "Male Menopause" but this is a misnomer for men have no "monthly periods." According to authorities the proper term should be "Andropause" connoting that the male hormone androgen has naturally declined.

The physical and psychological changes in andropausing male are manifested by: Loss of hair; testicles become smaller in size; decrease in muscular strength; low sperm count; decrease of bone density; and forgetfulness. Generally, there is a feeling of utter confusion, uncertainty, disillusionment and insecurity. A man of midlife crisis would appear with wrinkles on his face, eye bags, white hairs, receding hairline or balding, sagging skin, bulging stomach, poorer vision and hearing, fat and other veritable signs of aging. One has to realize that he has passed his peak in life and things have started to go downhill from then on.

However, things are not as bad as they seem to be. There is a positive after thought--"If there is life, there is hope." Hence, accept the unavoidable aging process and let go of whatever shortcomings or failures. One can still achieve some important goals and learn to enjoy the remaining years of his life by going through satisfactorily the aging period well.

Here are some meaningful activities suggested by this writer and people who went through the crisis and survived.

- Continue your health boosters: balance diet, regular exercise, anti-stress vitamins and minerals, etc.
- Understand yourself and be open to change.
- Stop vices-smoking, drinking, womanizing, etc.
- Rest and sleep well and learn to relax as you age.
- Form a good and profitable hobby of your choice.
- Pursue a life mission-community service.

- Share your wisdom and expertise by being a consultant or a mentor.
- Harness your creative talents in music, painting, writing, and join an art club and support groups or socio-civic organizations (if you are solvent).
- Search for wholesome activities and things that nourish your soul by being a spiritual person.
- Consult a specialist.

You can embrace age gracefully or fail! It is your choice, my friend.

Never Ignore any Severe Bleeding

In most normal situations, such as in tooth extraction or accidental cut by a sharp kitchen knife when slicing a vegetable, bleeding from a small wound blood clots within seconds or few minutes. However, in serious injuries or other disorders are involved, the body's normal blood-clotting function maybe inadequate or malfunctioning; if blood loss is not stopped, death may result.

Hemorrhage is the technical term for bleeding, often referring to substantial blood loss or uncontrollable bleeding externally or internally.

When the blood-clotting mechanism is temporarily inadequate (usually caused by serious injury) external hemorrhage results; when the blood-clotting mechanism has been disrupted as a result of some disorders (including hemophilia, peptic ulcer, cancer, kidney, or urinary tract) internal hemorrhage may result.

Severe external hemorrhage may result when a big blood vessel is cut (artery or vein) due to severe injury which happens in stab or open wounds, gunshots, or crushing accidents, etc. and which shows the following symptoms: rapid pulse, dizziness or faintness; collapse; shock; a drop in blood pressure; and pallor, cold clammy, or sweaty skin.

Internal hemorrhage may also show symptoms, even if the bleeding is slight. For instance, black, tarry stools may signal bleeding in the upper intestinal tract from a peptic ulcer or cancer of the colon; bleeding in the lower gut like the lower colon or rectum may show fresh blood; blood in the vomitus indicates bleeding in the stomach and blood in the urine means bleeding occurring in the kidneys or urinary tract. However, after a severe trauma, like falling from a deep ravine but no external sign of bleeding, the doctor will still observe the victim's condition in the hospital for a possible internal hemorrhage such as bleeding in any of the organs like spleen, pancreas, kidney, etc. and the encapsulated organ may just burst suddenly and hemorrhage may result and may cause untimely death.

Treatment for external bleeding is easier to manage when one knows First Aid by immediately putting a tourniquet or applying pressure on the bleeding point or wound with a sterile bandage (or, in an emergency, just pressing it with the fingers until the bleeding stops). If bleeding cannot be stopped, rush the patient to the hospital where lost blood can be replaced by blood transfusion and damaged blood vessels can be surgically tied off and sealed.

In the case of cerebral bleeding as shown by CT scan, the victim must be seen by a neurosurgeon, who will open a hole (trephining) in the brain, suck by a suction pump the accumulated blood and suture the damaged blood vessels and thus stopping the bleeding. Doctors usually prescribe Vitamin K (Ex. Hemostan Capsule) to stop the smaller internal bleeding. He should know the specific cause of the bleeding and treat it permanently.

Nervous Tension and Its Management

*"In the entire world, the
unhappiest creature is man."*
Anatole France

It is a fact that there is no time in our lives when we are completely happy. We have always had to worry over the lot of work, school, indebtedness, getting enough food to eat, having shelter over our head, whether we can still survive the next strong natural catastrophes–– typhoons, earthquakes, tsunamis, conflagrations, and other stressful activities in life.

There are times when we would like to escape from the tensions and turmoil of everyday living. But our conscience does not permit us to do so. So we often pay a high price in suffering from nervous tension.

Here are some signs of tension:

- Feeling of uneasiness or restlessness
    Ex. Habitual teeth-gritting, lip-tightening, nail-biting, pain at the nape
- Getting no satisfaction from life's small joys; a humorless life
- Being suspicious of people and mistrustful of friends
- Getting intensely angry at small irritations
- Being chronically tired; no pep at all
- Finding hard to sleep or rest

- Easily forgetful, absent-mindedness
- Oversensitivity; an onion skin, untouchable
- Hypertension

When tension becomes intolerable, it eventually leads to a psychological illness called **"psychosomatic responses"** such as gastric ulcer, high blood pressure, bronchial asthma, impotence, migraine, headache, obesity, etc.

How to manage tension
(There are relaxing ways to relieve tension.):

1. It is always beneficial to verbalize or express one's inner (unresolved) feelings or conflicts. Never pint-up or repress your feelings. Talk it out with a trusted friend.
2. Working off tension through exercising, jagging, punching a bag, walking, etc.
3. Take a worthwhile vacation, seeing a nice movie; take a cold or warm bath; have a relaxing massage; listen to soothing music.
4. Seek a professional help if things are unbearable.
5. Pray for enlightenment.

Suicide: A preventable Death

*"Often the test of courage is
not to die but to live."*
Conti Vitterie Alfieri

Among people, the word "suicide" commonly connotes different less serious implications. In daily usage a lot of persons casually express suicide to mean: "I'll go ahead and take the risk." *"Bahala na"* (come what may); to an avid gambler, it could mean, "I'll bet this game win or lose." But to a bad *politician-"siguradong mananalo ako* (I'll win) for I have goons, guns and gold. No need for suicide for he already lives comfortably in "hell" (hell side).

Let us now focus on the serious meaning of suicide. Apparently, most people are appalled when they hear that someone has committed suicide. Definitely, suicide is a gruesome way to die. Questions are always raised. Why? What happened? And so on and so forth. Each victim has his/her own story to tell (if he/she still lives after an attempt). Most often than not, an episode of depression is always behind the self-destructive process. The victim is said to be suffering from an affective (mood) disorder.

As to its prevalence, it is estimated that in an adult population, 3% is believed to have committed suicide. The incidence of suicide before was common among the elderly. However, the picture today has drastically changed because at the present time, suicide is apparently increasing among the younger aged group involving the adolescence from 15 to 19 years old. Suicide attempts generally are related to depression, alcoholism and drug dependency. Elderly males with serious chronic illness have greater risk of suicide.

Statistics show that persons who truly possess a very strong faith and practice his spiritual program consistently well are less prone to resort to self-destructive process. But, however, being "religious," as researchers discovered, will <u>never</u> prevent anyone from committing suicide. Reports abroad have confirmed that even some priests, ministers and a bishop have already committed suicide. Cause: their <u>seronin</u> level dropped too low.

Management. When anyone discovers that a certain person is planning to commit suicide, then, watch him very closely and keep away all potential deadly objects (i.e. ropes, wires, knives, poisonous solutions, guns, etc.)

Refer him/her to any psychiatrist for treatment. (Hospitalize him or put him on close watch at home.) The doctor can prescribe <u>antidepressants</u> and give psychotherapy to finally resolve the deep seated conflicts which cause the miserable depression.

Anyone who commits this "Judas Complex" is tantamount to <u>jumping to hell</u>-for only the Creator--God, can take the life of his creatures. Those who negates this truth is already doomed! Never gamble your only life, man. Otherwise, you burn in the Lake of Fire-forever.

The Amazing Technology of Cataract Microsurgery

Cataract is one of the most common eye afflictions of man. The real cause of cataract is unknown. Aging may play a role in its development. However, newborns whose mothers contacted German measles during pregnancy and some young people may also develop the condition.

The term **cataract** is from the Greek word for **waterfall** because people with it see their environment as if they are looking through a waterfall.

Cataract is the disease of the lens of the eye producing progressive deterioration of vision leading up to blindness. The definitive cure for this disease is surgical removal of the opaque lens and the implantation of a new intraocular lens.

Most competent and experienced surgeons have a 99% success rate. The microsurgery is painless, bloodless, and takes only few minutes to finish.

Symptoms of Cataract–– blurring of vision occurring most often in one eye. Then the other eye also follows or deteriorates (blurred). The patient may experience glare in bright light.

Precaution for People with Hypertension

Admittedly, a lot of people with high blood pressure are unaware of the factors that would trigger of an attack of hypertension. Medical authorities report claims that hypertension is a "silent killer." Many people have suddenly died of high blood pressure without knowing the real and immediate cause.

Here are ways to prevent the sudden attack of hypertension.

1. Be sure to check your blood pressure regularly.
2. Know the common causes of high blood pressure.
    Ex. High cholesterol diet, saturated fatty foods, too salty foods, etc.
3. Avoid being too emotional like sudden outburst of anger.
4. On the stairways of high-rise buildings–– always walk, never run.
5. Try to get a nap at least twice a day.
6. Remember to quit before you get so tired.
7. Avoid heated arguments.
8. A little outdoor exercise is beneficial.
9. Be weight conscious.
10. Be moderate in all your activities in life.

11. Know the principles of stress management.
12. Shun the type "A" personality. Be a man of good will.

Attitude Towards Aging and Getting Old

Most people could not differentiate between aging and getting old. Well, it's more than just the spelling. For people who possess positive outlook in life, healthy aging involves some characteristics feature

1. The person should have a positive attitude towards life.
2. He should know how to avoid getting diseases and injuries.
3. He should have a good health-promoting behavior (Ex. No bad habits and vices).
4. He should know the skills of stress management.
5. He should know how to handle problems and challenges that come his way. In other words he should know "how to roll with the punches."

Successful Aging is synonymous to full maturity, a period in life where one has reached his actual potential or personal fulfillment.

Getting Old means the belief that the person has reached the point of extreme passivity, boredom, and weakness.

1. The person has lost interest in life.
2. He develops the notion that it's too late to change.
3. He fails to make goals and commitments.
4. He loses the sense of surprises.

Essential Factors to be Observed in the Aging Process

Inevitably, man grows older every minute in a day without knowing it. He only realizes that aging is beginning to creep in his mind and body because his memory is no longer sharp; he misses to name his children, respectively. In doing his physical activities, he feels some aches and pains in his body, so much so that he begins to be extra careful in his movements and doing his daily routines.

Authorities suggest some useful activities that would help minimize the pangs of growing old. Here are some suggestions.

1. Observe proper diet, exercise, enough rest and sleep.
2. Continue doing your wholesome activities in life.
3. Do things in moderation.
4. Refrain from vices and bad habits like smoking, drinking and drug abuse.
5. Don't let your emotions rule you; like useless anxiety, anger and heated arguments.
6. Seek early medical assistance from proper authorities for any health problem.
7. Cultivate a prayerful and strong spiritual life.

Know Top Anti-Cancer Food Elements

Nutrition authorities report that cancer or malignant neoplasm rate is increasing throughout the world.

A book entitled "Beating Cancer with Nutrition" by Dr. Patrick Quillin, PhD., an American nutritionist and researcher, tells the readers about the natural ways to prevent cancer.

Here are some of the major sources of food elements that contain the necessary nutrients or anti-cancer properties to fight malignancy or cancer.

1. VEGETABLES: colorful beets, spinach, carrots, tomatoes, squash, etc. The deeper the color the more phytochemical, bioflavonoid and carotenoids. They contain anti-oxidants that destroy cancer cells.
    Cabbage Family-broccoli, cauliflower, brussel sprouts, etc.
    Alliums Family-onion and garlic.
2. COLD WATER FISH: ex. tuna and fish from the deep ocean contain Omega-3 and other fish oil from salmon, etc.
3. LEGUMES: like garbanzos, kidney beans, pinto beans, etc. They contain soluble fibers, etc.
4. WHOLE GRAIN: wheat, barley, rice, com, oats, etc.
5. KELP: "Sea vegetables or seaweeds" with many traces of minerals.
6. YOGURT: with lactobacillus ferments, protects our gastrointestinal tract.
7. GREEN TEA: catechins and other phytochemical with good cancer fighting agents.
8. HEALTHY SEASONING: like garlic, onions, mustard, curry, pepper, cinnamon, and ginger. They contain immune stimulating elements.
9. GRAPEFRUIT JUICE: contains powerful anti-cancer medicine known as "rapamycin" which stops the growth of new blood vessels where cancer tumor likes to grow.
10. DRINKING WINE: is beneficial in fighting

against Hodgins Lymphoma, a common lymph node cancer.

11. WALNUT: is found to have anti-cancer property.
12. CLEAN WATER: provides a healthy flow of nutrients into the cells and eliminates toxins out of the body cells.

Most of these food elements are available in our groceries and markets. So, make a list and be sure to buy them as part of your personal anti-cancer prevention diet. Eating more of the above enumerated foodstuffs will fortify you from getting sick with deadly cancer.

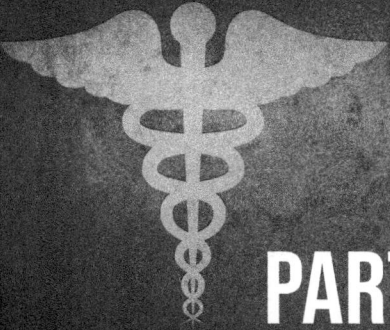

PART III

NEGATIVE BEHAVIOR TRAITS NOBODY WANTS

Procrastination-The Thief of Time

> *"Procrastination is a villain that can thwart our ambition, destroy our happiness, even kills us!*
>
> Norman Vincent Peale

Admittedly, one of the worst negative traits of many Filipinos is procrastination. We are fond of delaying or postponing an important action. A motto of procrastinators: *"Do not do today, what you can do tomorrow."* Definitely, this is a lazy man's belief that consequently leads to detrimental repercussions. Procrastination, once it becomes well-ingrained in our character is so difficult to cure. So let us nip into the bud before it grows into a monstrous proportion and impossible to manage.

Let us try to understand the psycho-dynamics of procrastination. Edward R. Dayton, an American lecturer and author of books on Time Management, explains the possible causes of procrastination. He claims that people procrastinate and fail to act most of the time because it is basically due to fear. He observes that people are afraid to be evaluated; afraid they will make a mistake and be criticized by others; afraid the result will not be perfect. He further says that people are afraid that they are not the ones to make the decision and are just to be ignored. Sometimes, we are afraid of completing the job and wonder what to do next. And we vacillate what to do first. So, we delay our action.

We can just imagine the numerous "sins of omissions" that one has committed in one's life. How many lives were littered with promises that were never kept, resolutions that were never fulfilled, intentions that were never honored, appointments and meetings that did not happen? We tend to push everything into tomorrow–– and tomorrow never comes.

Consider the following painful consequences of unnecessary postponements. How many people died because of putting off in going to the doctor early? How many houses of buildings were totally burned because the owners failed to notify the Fire Dept. of a faulty electric wire that sparks occasionally? How many people became victims of landslides or their houses were swept away by raging water but were waiting much earlier to transfer long before the calamity happened? How many marriages have been disintegrated because irresponsible couples failed to fulfill their sacred vows? Or, how many intelligent students failed to graduate because they preferred first to enjoy the pleasurable pursuits in life than to be serious in their studies?

And so many other important events and promising circumstances in life that utterly failed because of "manana habit" of people. They must have realized this faulty trait but probably, because of their inherent indolence and love of pleasures have prevailed in their lives and thus became the perennial procrastinators.

Here are some steps as suggested by expert authorities:

- Regard procrastination as a very serious problem.
- One must exert so much effort to stave off this bad trait.
- Strongly discipline yourself especially matters of <u>time</u> and effort.
- Make a list of your priorities for the day and do them consistently one by one until all are finished, no matter how hard. No excuses please.
- Don't be a perfectionist or too meticulous. This behavior wastes so much time.
- Conquer procrastination once and for all. It is really a very destructive habit, mind you.

No doubt, most people who are happy are those who have conquered the chains of procrastination. Why? They have fully satisfied doing their job on time well. They are full of eagerness, zest and productivity. Most of them are successful in life.

A short prayer for procrastinators-"Lord, may I do the things I should do, and may I find time for the things I want to do for your greater honor and glory."

Kleptomania

Parents were shocked and ashamed when their child was discovered and caught stealing things from friends and classmates. The reporting teacher could hardly believe that it was happening to a child of well-known, prominent parents in the community. The attention of the parents was called by the office and so it became the talk of the town, because of the ignorant people who are only good in their "Hitachi" business: *Hi-himantayon* (observant); *Ta-tabian* (talkative); *Chi-chismosa* (gossiper) and will wag their tongues and do their demolition job.

What is really Kleptomania?

Kleptomania is a psychiatric disorder and is defined as compulsive stealing of things of no real intrinsic value, not needed for personal use or their monetary value. This means that the Kleptomaniac steals objects or things that have no value to him or her. Psychoanalysts claim that a Kleptomaniac steals things that have sexual attachment like bracelets, rings, towels, stockings or lingerie. Kleptomaniacs are easily caught when they go to Department Stores to steal or shoplift. (Unlike the real robbers who steal for financial gains. They are the sociopaths or the criminally inclined. They steal money, hold-up people and rob banks.)

Kleptomaniacs grow up in families whose parents are quite seductive and with exhibitionistic tendency. Their children are neglected from the tender-loving-care of the parents. The act of stealing is a "call-for-attention device as well as an outlet for sexual craving."

For people with such a behavior, psychiatric help is imperative.

Sadism and Masochism

Admittedly, there are strange or queer behaviors of man that baffles us in this world. Sadism and masochism are such behavioral traits that are too shocking and could hardly be believed by conservative people.

Sadism is a form of sex perversion in which the loved one must be tortured; the erotic thrill is derived from cruelty, while **masochism** is sexual stimulation through passively enduring pain. Psychoanalysts claim that the two behavioral traits go hand in hand, hence the term sadomasochism-meaning that the sadist could also be a masochist. Normally they are a perfect team. But sadomasochism should be coupled with genuine love and tenderness to achieve genuine love-making.

In a hotel, a sadist staying in a room was heard saying, "Let me beat someone today!" In the adjacent room a masochist heard his plea and answered loudly saying, "Let it be me!!!"

Sexual sadism is the most common form of deviation in our society today. Our young lovers are indulging in heavy petting. This "love bites" is a form of sadistic kiss on the neck of the girl known as "chickenini," and this forces the girl to wear turtleneck even during summer months. Sadistic husbands are fond of painfully squeezing the delicate cells of the mammary glands of their wives, thus causing destructive changes like cancer.

Moral masochism is exemplified by the flagellants in Pampanga every Lent. They allow themselves to be nailed on the cross to expiate for their sins-popular Tourist Attraction.

Parents, managers, and individuals who are cruel and use violence are said to be sadists.

Seek for a professional help before it's too late.

Gossip--The Verbal Violence

*"The dog has many friends
because the wag was put in his
tail instead of in his tongue."*
Anonymous

Unfortunately, we have to admit that many of our folks are now caught in a web of what we call "tongue-mongering" (gossiping). They love to listen to malicious talks and savor its negative influences and its power to corrupt. Gossip is unconsciously used as a defense mechanism of the attacker's sense of inadequacy and helplessness--sort of a "counter punch" towards those whom they hate and envy.

Gossipers do not have qualms of conscience. It shows their weak character and are known as verbally sadistic. They love to spread rumors and viciously damage reputations of innocent and defenseless people. A study on Psychology of Rumor, Dr. Gordon Alport concluded that "as rumor travels, it grows shorter and more concise and becomes more easily grasped and told."

Since gossip is usually communicated in private and offered without proof, a victim of gossip is powerless against its ruthlessness. A writer in the New City magazine, Rene C. de Jesus says that "Gossip is considered to be pernicious it happens in the workplace for it creates so much havoc in terms of loss of productivity, and wasted times, low morale, heightened anxiety, suspiciousness and divisiveness among employees.

Gossip is now regarded as a form of "workplace violence." It is a character assassination of helpless workers.

Every religion in the world definitely considers gossip as evil. Let us quote some excerpts from the Holy Bible.

"Do not spread slanderous gossip among your people." (Leviticus 19:16, NLT); "He who repeats a matter alienates a friend." (Proverb 17:9 RSV); "There words are like an open pit and their tongues are good only in telling lies." (Roman 3:13 CEV); "Tattlers are spreading things which they ought not." (1 Timothy 5:13, KJV). According to St. Phillip, "It is impossible to gather gossip back once it comes out of our mouth." Here is an old adage worth remembering: "He who gossips to you will also gossip about you." So, never trust a gossiper.

As authentic Christians, we are expected to do our share of respecting and not participating in the cruel assassination of the person's character. We can choose to nip gossip in the bud by politely suggesting that we don't want to talk bad about someone who is not present to defend himself/herself. This gesture will show our clear stand against gossip. The gossipers will learn that we will never listen to nor spread gossip. They will realize that we are a truly trustworthy people. We will not jeopardize ourselves by using our untamed and vile tongue as a major instrument that will bring us to hell!

Dishonesty

(The Significance of Spiritual Health)
"The function of wisdom is discriminating between good and evil."

Cicero

A truly wise and "smartest" Christian must truly discern the priceless value of SPIRITUAL HEALTH which is more than gold and treasure the "pearl of Great Price," as Christ said. Undoubtedly, as an authentic Christian, this is our greatest goal in life, according to Anne Graham Lotz, the daughter of evangelist Billy Graham. The primary purpose of our existence in this world is not to achieve a healthy body, material riches, fame, power, etc. but to "ADORE and THANK GOD IN ALL HIS GLORY!" God created us in His own image and wanted us to live with Him for all Eternity in Heaven (that is if we truly follow His Commandments.)

However, the problem of man is his great tendency to follow his own free well and gravitate to the level of least resistance always towards pleasurable pursuits in life and readily would rationalize "sapagkat tao lamang ako." (I am just human.) He ignores and does not fully realize the fact that his physical existence is only transitory and the inevitability and unpredictability of death faces him every moment. Of course, man has free choices but he does not care about the outcome of his act–– "Bahala na!" (Come what may.)

As long as man is alive, he usually gives importance mostly to his body but not as much to his spiritual welfare. Someone said: "The way to hell is always paved with good intentions." Satan is so smart, indeed. He wins all the time (or most of the time).

An American clergyman, Rev. Fr. Robert Roleiser, once spoke about the "Spirituality of Commitment." He cited that in John's Gospel, there is a sin against the Holy Spirit. What is this sin? It is the sin of lying, the cover up, grave dishonesty. The good clergy said that all sins can be forgiven, but if you sin, don't lie about it. Hell begins here...a life (habit) of lying and corruption. The great lesson is–– if we want to go to Heaven, then, we don't have to lie! We have to live a life of transparency–– a genuine life of honesty and integrity. The reward of truth is the inner peace and joy. The Holy Bible says:

"The truth shall set you free." (Luke 8:30 KJV) Hence, we must vow to stop lying in our life. This is the greatest challenge to all the Filipinos who are deeply wallowing in the mud of corruption and dishonesty–– all extremely grave spiritual ill-health.

We fervently pray to Almighty God to always protect us from this evil and spare us from His devastating punishments. We have been fairly warned, and so let us change our wicked ways before it's too late.

Workaholic Syndrome

"Over-ambitious people frenzied themselves to work by burning their candles on both ends, unknowingly taxing their hearts to early death!"

Anonymous

Every living creature on earth knows the value of work for survival. Moderate work, as Thomas Carlyle says, is the grand cure of all the maladies and miseries that ever beset mankind. My late father, Alejandro, used to remind his growing children about the essence of work by quoting an old English saying, "He who does not work, shall not eat."

A lot of people may not be too aware that working beyond their normal capacity can lead to severe strain (stress) on their heart vessels that causes a fatal heart attack. The most vulnerable age groups, as reported by studies, are the young and middle-aged adults (prime of life). These are the ambitious hard-driving people who always work overtime day and night, burning candles at both ends to get rich quick. This is commonly known as "workaholism" or psychiatrists term as "Workaholic

Syndrome." The personality make-up is described to be a person who is overambitious, the hurrying kind who is addicted to work.

Two well-known American psychologists -Dr. Meyer Friedman and Dr. Ray H. Rosenman reported a fascinating research some years ago on the correlation between the personality type and coronary disease in their book-"Type A Behavior and Your Heart." This book concerns about the hard-driven person who becomes readily a victim (proneness) of heart attack (i.e. coronary thrombosis or artery disease, myocardial infarction).

Here are some major attitudinal characteristic features of a typical Workaholic or Type "A" personality:

- When one is always in a hurry; talking and walking rapidly; constantly looking at his watch; and worrying about being late.
- If one feels guilty when he is relaxing and doing nothing for several hours or a number of days.
- When one does not have any more time for vacation and leisure.
- If upon meeting another person, one feels compelled to compete with him.
- If one's work has caused him to suffer symptoms of stress such as headaches, bodily pains, hypertension, and fatigue.
- When one quantifies everything and finds himself evaluating not only his own but also the activities of others.
- When one attempts to schedule more and more in less and less time and unable to say no to people who want his services.
- When one is no longer interested in things that used to give him pleasure.

- When one's relationship suffers because he is always busy, too hurried, and put projects above people and mostly missing the company of his wife, children and friends. And finally, his wife says-"I'm missing my husband all the time...," "He has no real friends."

YOU ARE A CLASSICAL WORKAHOLIC and a strong candidate for Heart Attack!

The roots cause of his behavior could be traced to ambitious parents who unduly push their children to succeed and force them to compete and excel in school and outside and to conduct their affairs more quickly and aggressively than others.

The most beneficial management suggests changing Type "A" to Type "B" (a moderate lifestyle) may still lengthen and improve the quality of their lives. To cure this *"Hurry Sickness"* is to follow the Relaxation Therapy advocated by clinical therapists.

Change their lifestyle to protect them from heart attack or stroke. Have a healthy diet (low cholesterol), regular exercise, avoid smoking and achieve a consistent spiritual program in life.

Anger/Hostility-Taming the Beast in Us

*"It is better to put out the fire
when it's in the basket than
when it's racing up the wall."*
Dr. Steve Harper, PhD

Normally, everyone from childhood to old age has experienced getting angry when one's temper and emotion becomes inflamed. Anger is one of the most common and powerful emotions of man.

Psychoanalysts define **anger** as a spontaneous feeling of rage when one's right is trampled upon or transgressed. This is also known as **righteous anger.** This is exemplified when our Lord Jesus Christ got terribly mad when the money changers made the temple or church as a market place. Christ not only shouted at them but He got a cord and whipped them. However, after the confrontation, He calmed down and admonished them, like a good parent and became friendly again-- no rancor of hearts.

The social anthropologist, Konrad Lorenz, considers anger as a primary aggressive behavior of man with the intention to do physical and psychological harm directed towards people, objects, or self.

Hostility, on the other hand, is defined as an unresolved anger with a secret motive for revenge. It is a persistent anger as a result of frustrations. The best example of hostility is the strong unresolved anger of Adolf Hitler against the Jews who ransacked the German economy. He ordered millions of Jews killed in the gas chamber.

We have to discern the difference between the healthy and destructive anger. Generally, anger is aroused either by fear, hurt or frustration. These are emotional pains triggered by being insulted, ignored, rejected, deceived, and provoked.

We need to understand how damaging anger can be. Intense and unreasonable anger can sometimes lead to murder, such as uncontrolled crimes of passion.

Anger has been linked to hosts of health problems from anxiety, high blood pressure, bleeding peptic ulcers, heart attack, stroke, stress to drug and alcoholic abuse. Researchers have found that women who suppress anger have higher breast cancer rates and unhappy marriages and are two times likely to die prematurely than those who directly expressed their anger. And hostile men who flare-up uncontrollably their anger are likely to die suddenly to cardiovascular diseases.

Psycho-social and spiritual authorities suggest sound advices on how to quench the unpredictable fury and better handle anger by the following proven effective measures:

- Just pray a flash prayer-"arrow prayer" (i.e. repeating parts of the gospel verses, say, "Make haste to help me, O Lord" or "God create a clean heart in me."
- Dissipate anger in socially acceptable ways. Do nothing. Think clearly. Just keep quiet. Don't add fuel to the fire. Speak calmly.
- Control your wrath no matter how serious.
- Leave the tense scene for a while.
- Cool off, take a shower, beat a pillow, and scream in a closed room.
- When things are calm, ask for forgiveness.
- Be sensible, control your temper.
- Seek professional help to finally resolve conflicts.
- If you can't handle anger, then anger will certainly destroy you.

Now, if things will still don't work and your life is truly endangered, then call the authorities, barangay (barrio) captain or police to rescue you and have your case documented or blottered, okay?

Forgetfulness

*"The true art of memory is
the art of attention."*
Samuel Johnson

How many of us have experienced forgetting the name of a friend just when you were about to introduce him to other friends? Or you were forced to turn back home while on the road because you're not sure whether or not you shot off the appliance? Or, you were frustrated of not knowing where you place your car keys while you were about to go home from shopping. Well, these are just temporary bouts of forgetfulness, but have already stressed you so much. However, it does not mean you are completely losing your memory.

Psychologists claim that our ability to recall things should remain sharp well into our sixties. Although natural changes occur with the memory process as we age and there is no cause for alarm for forgetfulness is curable for normal people.

Of course, severe cerebral damage involving our brain cells, vessels, and nerves as in Alzheimer's disease, atherosclerosis in old age (senile changes), and other brain injuries due to alcoholism, drugs, etc. which cause a steady deterioration of brain tissue functions will produce a continuing loss of memory. However, brain specialists optimistically claim that "no matter what your age is, you can still improve your memory."

Your memory is like any muscle-the more it is exercised, the stronger it becomes. Here are some time-proven suggestions for keeping your memory in good shape. So, train your brain to remember and always keep focus.

- Keep calm. Stress and anxiety can disrupt memory performance. You need your serene consciousness to encode things. Anxious people are forgetful or absent-minded.
- Always pay attention and fully concentrate. Don't be a scatter-brain. Avoid any distractions.
- Make meaningful connections. Associate a story or a sentence that links on information in a meaningful way. Invent your own reminders (i.e. use some "formula or acronyms." Example: "T.L.C.-Tender Loving Care.")
- Paint a mental image. Concrete visual image can help you connect new names and faces.
- Review what you want to remember. Repetition is essential to make a deeper mental tract in the memory center of your brain.
- Think and look for any distinct "markers" or cues or sign that could lead or tip-off your memory.
- Organize what you know into a meaningful pattern. Make a well-kept filling system where things are easily found.
- The best time to memorize is before bedtime and immediately after rising early in the morning.
- Keep your mind clean and safe from artificial and destructive elements.

Never forget to pray to the Holy Spirit for a superb memory. You'll never regret it!

Shyness

*"In my shyness, I was afraid
to speak or be noticed.
I sat alone for hours and kept silent.
I was afraid of my own shadow."*

Anonymous

Generally, Filipinos are known to be shy people or *"mahiya-in"* in the vernacular. If shyness will be carried too far and cannot be stopped, certainly, this negative trait will lead to a miserable and stressful existence of shyness. This trait of extreme bashfulness has been attributed to our culture or family upbringing. Most Filipino mothers usually instill in the minds of their children to be always humble, modest, unpretentious, unassuming, and to be quiet. This is because to be *"manghambog"* (to show off) you put the whole family to shame. Another significant factor is the influence of our religious belief-"Be humble and meek of heart" to be pleasing to God. Remember, "Pride goes before the fall". It is the No. 1 cardinal sin as pious people would say.

Most unfortunate victims of shyness are the oversensitive individuals who are suffering from physical defects like cross-eyed or squint, hare-lip, limping, ugly-looking as well as those stubborn and rebellious or disobedient children who are always subjected to criticisms and ridicules by cruel parents or bad people. It could also be caused by heredity.

Shyness is the unpleasant feeling that forces a person to withdraw from people because of the negative thoughts that dominate his mind. It is synonymous to timidity or bashfulness. It is a psychologically handicapping trait. One becomes extremely withdrawn, a loner, and an outcast in society.

The psychodynamics of shyness–– Shyness causes intense self-personal pre-occupation with one's thoughts, feelings and reactions. It causes an extremely uncomfortable feeling and also inhibits interpersonal relationship as well as interferes with pursuing one's professional goals. Shyness, if not treated, would lead to a more serious condition as social phobia, an extreme withdrawal from social activities and people.

Here is a remarkable example of a person who conquered his extreme shyness and bashfulness. As a boy, he was too thin and painfully shy. But through the constant counsel of his professor in his sophomore year, he finally changed his shyness and became a foremost speaker and famous writer in the world. The boy's name was Norman Vincent Peale.

Today, psychoanalysts found Cognitive Behavioral Therapy (C.B.T.) as the best modality that works effectively. The therapist helps the client to change incorrect perceptions into rational and accurate thinking.

Guilt Feelings

"True guilt can be a healthy stimulant, a quick painful jolt to make us change."
Martin R. Padova

In College Literature, we learned about a serious example of guilt complex manifested by the "washing mania of Lady Macbeth," one of Shakespeare's tragedies. The Lady tried to repress her guilt feeling of murder but unconsciously she was relentlessly tortured and was forced to compulsively wash her hands several times a day to ritualistically remove her guilt. "I saw spots of blood in my hands!" (Guilty conscience.)

Generally, people with the right conscience have experienced the unpleasant feeling of guilt when they commit a serious culpable act. The Oxford Encyclopedic Dictionary defines guilt as "Fact of having committed a specified or implied offense."

So often, a man of scrupulous conscience can get so lock up into his past; what he did, what he said, the events of which he was ashamed of and made him to suffer mental anguish if he was not able to expiate for his serious misdeed. As Shakespeare quips, "Conscience makes coward of us all." An unresolved serious offense can torture a morally straight person in his entire life. This is like the "hound of heaven" that tracks us down like a criminal.

Psychologists say that genuine or true guilt is connected to wrongs we have done or good things we have left undone-"the sin of commission or omission." A certain Dr. Norman Buber said that the most poignant guilt stems from some violations of human relationship that cause us to say to ourselves "How could I have done that to him?" An existential or true guilt refers to a "positive and constructive emotion." True guilt arises from a violation of God's commandments. Such violations deliberate intentional acts that destroy or harm others and invoke real sense of guilt. A healthy conscience can serve to prevent the repeated commission of acts that evoke guilt-provoking behavior.

Psychiatrists have shown that the major cause of severe depression that leads to suicide is the unresolved chronic guilt that persistently tormented a person. We may call this as "The Judas Complex." Even the brilliant American writer Like Earnest Hemingway took his own life. The "neurotic" or unrealistic conscience could behave like a gestapo tracking down mercilessly trivial offenses committed even in dreams.

Guilt is believed to be a form of punishment. Punishing ourselves for past mistakes is an exercise of false pride. Let us free ourselves from guilt feelings by sincerely repenting, confessing and accepting God's forgiveness.

The Hypochondriac

"Imagination may be a blessing or a curse."

Oscar de Quiros

Intelligent and responsible individuals are expected to follow the rules of good hygiene and regular physical examination. But the hypochondriac is chronically over concerned with his body. He is a perpetual worrier.

Hypochondriasis is the persistent and exaggerated worry-usually based on self-diagnosis, an individual has about his or her health even though he or she is not actually ill. This term is originally thought to affect the region of the stomach believed to be the "Center of Melancholy or Sadness".

Hypochondria reflect an often morbid concern over any unusual physical or mental sensation or feeling. For example, to a hypochondriac, a headache indicates a brain tumor or Cancer; a cough has to mean tuberculosis; and a mole is sure to be cancerous. Despite test results and reassurances, the person is convinced that he is sick with serious illness.

Symptoms common among hypochondriacs are pain or discomfort in the stomach, chest, head or neck. They also complain of nausea, vomiting and belching.

Studies reveal that these symptoms become worse after the person receives expression of sympathy and concern from family members and friends. The hypochondriac often makes visits to doctors and use a number of non-prescription drug items.

Treatment: Psychotherapy is most useful intervention in this psychologically motivated illness. Otherwise, it is difficult to cure.

Accident Proneness

"Mishaps are like knives that either
serve or cut us as we grasp the blade."
James Russel Lowe!

Mass media reports that a large number of Filipinos suddenly die or get permanently crippled everyday due to accidents. As to the exact number of deaths, nobody can tell for our accuracy of reporting (as to statistics) is deplorably poor.

However, we are so much concerned as to the possible causes of accidents for most road accidents are commonly identified to be due mostly to drunken drivers or perhaps under the influences of drugs or reckless driving. But the question is <u>what makes some people prone to accidents</u> (or accident proneness)?

Psychologists define accident-proneness as the <u>high susceptibility to accidents.</u> Studies have shown that there are individuals who have a high tendency to be an "accident repeater", a predisposition common to some people as we call in our culture as "<u>disgraciado</u>". These persons often meet accidents such as easily bumped, run-over, cut, etc. (Of course, not hit by a lightning, or hit by a big fallen tree of which are pure accidents.)

Research authorities said that accident-proneness in some people is found to be secondary to <u>unresolved emotional problems</u> which tend to increase and individual's distractibility and preoccupation. Thus, in many cases, these unconscious negative feeling gives rise to behavior which interferes with, for example, the safe operation of machines and hidden feelings of hostility which predispose drivers to car accidents; apathy or depression may induce carelessness; tension and anxiety may interfere with one's bodily coordination and that's the reason why some persons become so clumsy.

Studies clearly showed that in industry, an estimated 88% of accidents show that a great number of people have <u>negative or dangerous attitudes</u> which increase the probability of an accident.

Attitudes which characterize accident-repeaters are: <u>impulsiveness, aggressiveness,</u> fatalism, intolerance of authorities and stress. Common <u>stressful factors contributing to accident-proneness</u> are such conditions as: infections, lack of sleep, malnutrition, severe <u>menstruation causing anemia, hypoglycemia causing faintness or dizziness and physically uncomfortable work environment</u> (i.e. lack of ventilation, noise, etc.), emotional instability <u>and extreme stressful conditions.</u>

Psychiatrists have found evidence of suicidal impulses-a need of self-punishment in accident-prone patients called "<u>purposive accidents.</u>" They hurt themselves "accidentally on purpose" (unconscious motivation).

Safe behaviors are solely the concern of <u>Safety Educators</u> (parents, teachers, police) which should begin early in child's life to cultivate responsible attitudes towards the development of safety behavior.

Pray always to your Guardian Angel to protect you as you travel through the turbulent gauntlets of this life. May the Almighty God spare you from crippling accidents, my friends.

Castration Complex

People may not be aware that one of the most frustrating interpersonal relationships is the presence of a perennial conflict irritant between couples or members of the family. This negative kind of a relationship is known as **castration complex.**

Psychoanalytically, castration complex means **penis envy of the female** (Freud). It is believed that the girls are envious of the boys because the latter (boys) have a powerful penile instrument (penis) while the former (girls) do not have. Hence, the girls are known to be castrated. Sigmund Freud signified castration as a psychologically like one whose head is being beheaded or cut-off. Hence, it is being applied to a wife whose husband could not talk, decide, or offer any decision as a castrated husband. The same description is when a wife calls her husband as **dumb** and **stupid.** Some couples survive with this kind of one-sided relationship; the husband becomes so silent, timid and obeys his dominant wife who always castrates him.

What are the possible consequences in this one-sided situation? If the concerned husband happens to be a **masochist** (loves to receive pain), he may just tolerate and resign with the painful ordeal in his life. However, if the husband is not a masochist and he cannot endure the humiliating treatment of his castrating wife, and he realizes his rightful position as the head of the family, and he has all the rights plus the essential self-esteem, then he might just rebel and separate from the extremely castrating and sadistic wife who tortures him all the time.

Castration complex is never welcome in a mutual and reciprocal marital relationship. There should be a peaceful and loving relationship between Christian couples to make marriage last to the end. Hence, castration complex should be stopped by all means. Nobody wants to live with a castrated (no balls) or headless husband.

The evil consequence of a real castration existing between warring couples is an extremely chaotic marriage. There is no more peace whatsoever. The castrating wife utilizes her vile words as her sword to cut or behead (castrate) the husband's head every time he fights her. For instance, she truly hurts his self-esteem (pride) or silences him by enumerating all his past misdeeds to prove his badness.

The poor husband would just rationalize that his wife is not the God who had already pardoned him of all his past offences in the Sacrament of Penance. What is the use of all his heartfelt prayers and strong faith, and hope for the forgiveness of sins, if he continues to commit sin!

Transsexualisms

When God created the world, He was sure He created a real man and woman and named them Adam and Eve; not Adam and "Steve."

Transsexualism is the strong desire of a boy or a girl, man or woman to be in the opposite sex. Today, there are men and women who like to change their sex roles. Psychiatrists refer this as Sexual Orientation Disorder. History tells that the main cause of transsexualism is the full identification of the boy with his own mother whom he is so attached with since childhood and the total rejection of a cruel father whom he hates so much, or the absence of an ideal father. The other factor is environmental. The effeminizing trait could also be reinforced by the presence of male homosexuals around who befriend and influence him.

A married female nurse narrates that her father-in-law is a "Cross-dresser" or a transsexual. He is a retired Army Captain. There are moments when he goes out at night with a woman's attire and drives his car alone, and seeks for a male mate. His family, after noticing his abnormal behavior, tries to stop him from such shameful negative behavior. But he vehemently says, "I'll die if you stop me from doing so."

The transsexuals are difficult to change because they are "ego-syntonic," meaning they feel fully satisfied with their behavior.

Recommendation:

Authorities advise them to undergo surgical intervention to transform them to become what they wish to become "women," or "men."

Warning:

Be honest to accept the negative result of being a transsexual.

What are Attitudes?

*"Attitude is of paramount importance
that we should know how to harness
and control this great secret power."*
Charles Simmons

Someone has said that our attitude controls our lives. Attitude, whether good or bad, continuously works for twenty-four hours a day. Every person reflects his particular kind of attitude he learned since childhood.

He shows this particular outlook or disposition towards various things, persons, and ideas. These reactions are called "attitudes."

Attitude is defined simply as a "frame of mind or a point of view." Let us take our positive and negative reactions toward things, persons or ideas. For example: Self-esteem is an attitude that each one of us holds about ourselves. Attraction is a positive attitude towards another person, and prejudice is a negative attitude often directed towards a certain person or group.

Psychosocial authorities believe that our attitude is a combination of affective (mood), behavioral, and cognitive (perception) reactions to an object based on relevant beliefs, images, memories and experiences. People commonly describe their attitude towards an object as––like, dislike, love, hate, admire, detest, etc.

Our attitude, authorities claim, can vary in strength or level of intensity along both positive and negative dimensions. In other words, we can react to something with positive effect or with negative effect, with what we call in psychiatric parlance as ambivalence (a mixed emotion of love and hate towards the same person), or with apathy and indifference. This attitudinal reaction is automatic, like a reflex action.

Psychologists found that individuals differ in the extent to which one reacts to a stimulus in strong positive or negative terms. It would be good if individuals would tend to react in a more <u>objective, non-evaluated ways but not judgmental.</u> However, the problem is that a lot of people are opinionated on the whole range of social, and political issues. (Remember, opinions are not facts.)

When national elections are approaching, people are confused as to whom to choose from their best candidates. Their choice will depend on several factors. However, a lot of Filipinos are still deprived of good and reliable information and may be swayed only on what they hear or see in the ads of which are most gimmickry.

We hope and pray our people will truly use their God-given prudence-a cardinal virtue and the secret of a win-win attitude.

The Sociopath

"An abuser is a wolf in sheep's clothing."
Anonymous

The paramount objective and issue of this article is to let our young Filipino women be aware of the existence of a person in our society who disguises as a *"good sheep"* but in reality, he is a ravishing wolf who abuses and destroys women.

The second major message is-Please do not embark on the "Sea of Matrimony" where there are no compass ever invented yet. So, always follow the wise counsels of your elders and experienced counselors to reassure you of a safer travel in this life. Otherwise, regret comes last.

The *sociopath* is actually an old term describing a male whose character is quite questionable. A modem term given to this guy is "Anti-social Personality Disorder." To many, he may look "O.K." to most people in society, or show "good behavior" externally––*"pasantos-santos lang"* (acting like a saint). However, if anyone goes against his wishes, he becomes vindictive. If he is married, his wife always suffer from a "Battered Wife Syndrome".

Today many wives are duly informed about the Family Code of the Philippines, which was based on the Canon Law of the Catholic Church of November 27, 1983.

Basically, individuals who are incapable of contracting marriage because of Psychological Incapacity-referring to the most serious cases of personality disorders. For instance:

- Those who lack sufficient use of reason (mentally ill or psychotic)
- The Anti-social Personality Disorder (Sociopaths or Criminally-inclined persons)
- If either party is below 18 years of age
- Marriage without consent of parents
- Marriage obtain by fraud
- Marriage by intimidation or undue influence
- Party sick with Socially Transmitted Disease (STDS)
- Total absence of utter love, affection, trust and respect
- Infidelity or unfaithfulness
- Either couple abandoned the family, children, and without mutual support or negligence
- Violence or acts dishonoring the family reputation or honor
- Perversion
- Alcoholism, Drug Addiction, etc.

- Abuser show no remorse of conscience or guilt feelings

The above manifestations are grounds for psychological incapacity it proven true. The Plaintiff or Defendant is unfit to comply with the essential obligation of marriage. Then, marriage is civilly annulled.

Jealousy-The Green-eyed Monster

"Jealousy lives upon doubts. It becomes madness or ceases entirely as soon as we pass from doubt to certainty."
L. Rochefoucauld

When I was a kid, I used to hear a song-"Jealousy". It runs in part: "Jealousy, night and day you torture me..." Well, I understood the real meaning of the word when I grew up.

We should admit that there are moments in our life when we get jealous. This usually happens when we are insecure that what we may possibly lose especially something we value to someone else. This is a normal reaction. We sometimes suffer the unpleasant feeling of resentment, helplessness and insecurity. Jealousy has been a normal part of our lives. Jealousy is a close cousin of envy.

Psychologists said that jealousy tends to develop in childhood when the mother-child relationship is found wanting. The child feels insecure that what he loves or desires might be lost or be taken away from him. These negative childhood experiences are the root causes of jealousy. This is one of the major reasons that many of the promising relationships were destroyed because of unfounded jealousies. This is quite common among suspicious (paranoid) husbands who manifest what we call pathological jealousy in psychiatry. This is an abnormal trait.

Jealousy is one of those feelings that a person will never get rid easily in one's life. There is always a tendency that we keep a constant watch over the possibility that someone better than us might intrude into our relationship. A husband will often be consumed by rage even when he suspects his charming wife for her possible infidelity. Constant doubts and mistrusts often lead to jealousy.

Here are some risky moves committed by too trusting and unwary couples: Often, they show qualities that easily entice the opposite sex. For instance, living far away from each other, being intelligent, talented, a good conversationalist, a smart and witty person with good sense of humor, a stunning physique, a good dresser, very popular, amiable and extremely kind, rich, helpful (caring) and a generous person and other "idealistic" traits that every man or woman strongly desires to possess. Also, a too-trusting attitude that both spouses may not believe in marital conjoined therapy or counseling. Shun the "bahala na" (come what may) attitude.

Some pointers to guard against disastrous jealousy:

- Couples to avoid being very close toward any opposite sex.
- Both must closely guard themselves falling into the tender-trap at any cost.
- Establish an unconditional love for each other, no matter what happens.
- Follow god's Commandments to the end.
- Always pray together and be at peace.

- Seek early professional counseling if conflicts cannot be controlled or resolved.
- Remember: "For the perverse person is abominable to the Lord." (Prov. 3:31-32 NKJV)

Aggressive Behavior

The most persistent sound which
reverberates through men's history
is the beating of drums."
Arthur Keestiev

Everyone living in a peaceful and gentle society upon hearing of a prominent person shot to death will certainly be shocked. Everyday, we read in various newspapers of people murdered by unknown assailants with several motives of killing.

Let us try to understand, therefore, the various factors involved in aggressive behavior, like violence. Sigmund Freud and Konrad Lorenz regarded aggression as an innate, instinctual motivation. Other psychoanalysts claimed that <u>aggression is always caused by frustration.</u>

Authorities define aggressive behavior <u>as an act that is intended to do physical or</u> psychological harm. Violence means the infliction of physical force on others. The factors that contribute to aggressive behavior include:

- Genetic factor. Hereditary transmission such as the presence of an abnormal XYZ chromosomes which predisposed some individuals to violent behavior. An example is Richard Speck who killed several American and Filipino nurses decades back.

- Brain injury affecting the Limbic System... the center that controls emotional behavior like fighting, rage, and violent assaults in humans. This could happen when irate parents uncontrollably hit their children's head causing a minimum brain injury.
- A family who experienced social and emotional deprivations during childhood and adulthood, thus causing absence of real love, affection, respect, peace and happiness. Extreme poverty breeds criminality.
- The link between drugs and alcohol and aggressive behavior is well established. These substances damage the brain which cause poor impulse control. Hence, drug abusers and alcoholics are ever sensitive, violent and homicidal in nature.
- Personality defect (i.e. Antisocial Personality Disorder)... a sociopathic lifestyle inclined to commit criminal behavior. This character lacks moral values and could easily kill any person. It starts as conduct disorder in childhood.
- Mass media influence. This carries a double-edged message emphasizing the evil lifestyle of distressed persons and description of crimes they commit in detail. Reporters write and exposed the negative traits of criminals showing them in print and TV media, videos, films, etc. depicting violent behavior. Children and gullible adults consciously and unconsciously will learn the negative behavioral pattern, the conditioning process.
- Environmental factors. Guns and other deadly

weapons are readily available where one could easily secure, legally or illegally.

- The grip of economic crisis. The common victims of hard times are the disgruntled poor who may be used by the striving and ambitious bedeviled middle class to carry their hidden evil scheme to silence the unwary citizen. This usually happens in big cities where lucrative deals are rampant.

Therefore, all well-meaning citizens in society must commit and earnestly find ways to help the downtrodden in their midst, known by Mahatma Gandhi, as "the Least, the Last and the Lost. And of course, with a vigilant and efficient law enforcers to prevent and solve crimes.

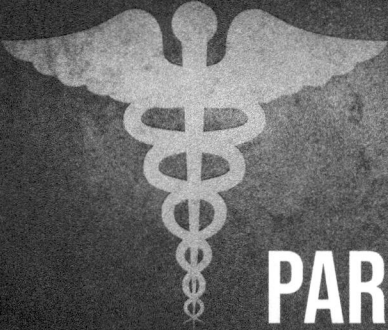

PART IV

PERSONALITY DISORDERS INDUCED BY EMOTIONAL FACTORS

The Neurotic Personality

This is a pattern of personality trait which renders the individual susceptible to an odd behavior characterized by a constant feeling of tension, apprehension, or prone to anxiety. The neurotic person is aptly described as oversensitive, or overemotional, overly cautious, fickle, meticulous, fanatical, too orderly individual who is likely to develop an obsessive-compulsive reaction as a strong defense maneuver. He is always **at edge** in life (too sensitive or over reactive).

Causes:

A. It is believe that the root cause of neurosis is basically the impaired parent-child relationship with parents who are harsh, overprotective and inconsistent.
B. The feeling of hidden inferiority due to some

obvious physical defect **(the ugly duckling complex).**

C. The strong sibling rivalry.
D. The morbid fear of punishment and rejection.
E. Mostly belonging to the struggling or middle class family.

Psychoanalysts say that neurotics have rigid superego (moralistic). How will they live and co-exist with the worldly or mundane people? Well, most of them use the protective defense mechanism of **sublimation and restitution** rechanneled their ID (sexual) drives. For instance, many of them join religious organizations and always preoccupy themselves with works or chores to deviate their strongly hostile mentality and other mundane thoughts. Many hold themselves to high standard of perfection; hence, they are deluded and become so hypercritical and cynical persons.

Neurosis highly affect more women than men. They are highly susceptible to stress and more prone to psychosomatic disorders.

Neurotic disorder is typically exemplified by the phobic individual who suffers from needless anxiety even though there is no immediate or real danger but present only in his imagination. In other words there is no realistic threat to his life. Other neuroticisms are manifested by the hysterical patients who dramatically display make-believe acts (faking) then their desires are not granted. We call this as **conversion reaction.**

In the Holy Bible, Jesus confronted a complaining woman: "Martha, Martha, you are a worrier about unimportant things! Mary has found a more important thing to listen to Jesus."

Psychiatrists have difficulty treating a neurotic than a psychotic patient!

Psychosomatic Illness

"The emotionally-caused illnesses make some doctors and quacks richer through their suggestions and patients' gullibility."
Anonymous

Probably, a lot of people know in everyday experience that fainting spells, blushing, pounding of the chest, tearfulness or crying, laughing, nausea or vomiting, etc. could be induced by emotional stimulation most especially to the easily suggestible, oversensitive or gullible individuals.

We have to know at the present moment that chronic or long-term emotional stress can promote or even set off long-term illness known as psychosomatic illness. Doctors often use the term to describe the illness induced by emotional or psychological factors.

The famous American Psychiatrist, Dr. Karl Menninger, estimated that half or 50% of the out-patients who consulted to doctors in their respective clinics suffered ailments related to unresolved inner conflicts in life such as fear, anger, resentment and other unresolved negative feelings. The human organism could no longer tolerate the constant and repeated stress and would therefore transfer the problem from the "psyche" (the mind) to the "soma" (the body). Hence, "psychosomatic" (mind-body) illness unconsciously would become meaningful to the affected organ of the person.

Psychosomatic illnesses that are induced by emotional factors are the following:

- Heart Attack-The expressions "heartbroken or died with a heavy heart."

- Peptic Ulcer-Victims are the "ambitious or aggressive, go-getter, independent type."
- Bronchial Asthma-Victims are the "oversensitive and allergic types of persons."
- Arthritic Patients-They are sensitive to life situations and have poor personal relationships.
- Hypertensive Patients-People who are unable to express their rage or anger.
- Impotence and Frigidity-Unresolved hostility towards the partner and sexual Ignorance.
- And many others--only psychiatrists can resolve them!

Antisocial Personality Disorder

Antisocial Personality Disorder was formerly known as Sociopathic Personality Disorder. The essential feature of this disorder is a pattern of irresponsible and antisocial behavior beginning in childhood or early adolescence and continuing into adulthood. For this diagnosis to be given, the person must be at least 18 years of age and have a history of Conduct Disorder before the age of 15.

Lying, stealing truancy, vandalism, initiating fights, running away from home, and physical cruelty are typical childhood signs. In adulthood the antisocial pattern continues, and include failure to honor financial obligations, to function as a responsible parent or to plan ahead, and an inability to sustain consistent work behavior. These people fail to conform to social norms and repeatedly perform antisocial acts that are grounds for arrest, such as destroying property, harassing others, stealing and having all illegal occupation.

People with Antisocial Personality Disorder tend to

be irritable and aggressive and to get repeatedly into physical fights and assaults, including spouse or child-beating. Reckless behavior without regard to personal safety is common, as indicated by frequently driving while intoxicated or getting speeding tickets. Typically, these people are promiscuous (defined as never having sustained a monogamous relationship for more than a year).

Finally, they generally have no remorse about the effects of their behavior on others; they may even feel justified in having hurt or mistreated others. After age 30, the more flagrantly antisocial behavior may diminish particularly sexual promiscuity, fighting and criminality.

Conclusion:

The Antisocial Traits will continue to exist to the adult life but may diminish after their late old age.

In the legal parlance, the Antisocial Personality Disorder is generally known as the "incorrigibles or the recidivists".

Schizotypal Personality Disorder

We all know that a human being is gregarious by nature from birth to death. A psychologically normal person always seeks for a partner or companion of for a group of persons or society where he could fit his ideas, his interests and capacities.

A schizotypal personality disorder person is compared to the queerest bird, the Owl because of his odd behavior; he likes to be alone, talk and laugh to himself. His ideas and beliefs are of his own imagination, so much so, that people cannot understand him.

The essential feature of this disorder is a pervasive

pattern of peculiarities of ideation, appearance and behavior and deficits in interpersonal relatedness, beginning by early adulthood and present in a variety of contexts that are not severe enough to meet the criteria for Schizophrenia.

The disturbance in the content of thought may include paranoid ideation, suspiciousness, ideas of reference, odd beliefs, and magical thinking that is inconsistent with subcultural norms and influences the person's behavior. Examples include supersticiousness, belief in clairvoyance, telepathy, or "sixth sense" or beliefs that "others can feel my feelings" (when it is not a part of a cultural belief system). In children and adolescents, these thoughts may include bizarre fantasies or preoccupations. Unusual perceptual experiences may include illusions and sensing the presence of force or person not actually present (e.g. "I felt an evil presence in the room"). Often speech shows marked peculiarities, but never to the point of loosening of associations or incoherence. Speech may be impoverished, digressive, vague, or inappropriately abstract. Concepts may be expressed unclearly or oddly, or words may be used in an unusual way. People with this disorder often appear odd and eccentric in behavior and appearance. For example, they are often unkempt, display unusual mannerisms, and talk to themselves.

Interpersonal relatedness is invariably impaired in this people. They display inappropriate or constricted effect, appearing silly and aloof and rarely reciprocating gestures or facial expressions, such as smiling or nodding. They have no close friends, or confidants (or only one) other than first degree relatives, and are extremely anxious in social situations involving unfamiliar people.

Associated features-Varying mixtures of anxiety, depression, and other dysphoric moods are common. Features of Borderline Personality Disorder are often present, and in some cases both diagnosis may be warranted. During period of extreme stress, people with this disorder may experience transient psychotic symptoms, but they are usually insufficient in duration to warrant an additional diagnosis. Because of peculiarities in thinking, people with Schizotypal Personality Disorder are prone to eccentric convictions.

Impairment-Some interference with social or occupational functioning is common.

Prevalence--Recent studies indicate that approximately 3% of the population has this disorder.

Sex ratio-No information.

Familiar pattern-There is some evidence that people with Schizotypal Personality Disorder are more common among the first-degree biologic relatives of people with Schizophrenia than among the general population.

Paranoid Personality Disorder

A. Definition.

People with this personality disorder exhibit a pervasive and standing suspiciousness and mistrust of people, hypersensitivity, hyper vigilance, unwarranted suspicions, jealousy, envy, and excessive feeling of importance, and a tendency to blame others and ascribe evil motives to them. They are regarded by others as hostile, stubborn and defensive. They may be litigious.

B. Features:

1. Persons with paranoid personalities rarely seek psychiatric treatment on their own.
2. The disorder is more common in men.
3. Most paranoid people avoid intimacy.

C. Etiology (cause).

Some think that paranoid personalities often have parents of the opposite sex who are domineering, overprotective, and ambivalent, and parents of the same sex who are submissive, passive and, as Freedman et al, wrote, relatively unavailable to the child "as an object for identification."

Generally, paranoid persons always claim without basis, what they believe on. Example:

1. A husband heard from a neighbor that his wife seated together and talking with a man in a bus going to the city. With this report the husband concluded that his wife has another lover.
2. At home, the parents have a lunch table conversation with some of their children. A son, who just arrived from school hears his name mentioned, thinks that they are talking something negative about him.

Management:

Paranoid personality disorder is beyond psychiatric intervention because this is deeply ingrained personality trait since childhood.

May God help him!

Histrionic Personality Disorder

The essential feature of this disorder is a pervasive pattern of excessive emotionality and attention seeking, beginning by early adulthood and present in a variety of contexts. In other classifications this category is termed Hysterical personality. People with this disorder constantly seek or demand reassurance, approval, or praise from others and are uncomfortable in situations in which they are not the center of attention. They characteristically display rapid shifting and shallow expression of emotions. Their behavior is overly reactive and intensely expressed; minor stimuli give rise to emotional excitability. Emotions are often expressed with inappropriate exaggeration, for example-the person may appear much more sad, angry, or delighted than would seem to be warranted. People with this disorder tend to be very self-centered, with little or no tolerance for the frustration of delayed gratification. Their actions are directed to obtaining immediate satisfaction.

These people are typically attractive and seductive, often to the point of looking flamboyant and acting inappropriately. They are typically overly concerned with physical attractiveness. In addition, their style of speech tends to be expressionistic and lacking in detail. For example, a person may describe his vacation as "Just Fantastic!" without being able to be more specific.

Histrionic Personality Disorder is common to Movie Stars or Movie Actresses. Watch them behave, talk, act with their respective role plays; how they dress attractively and seductively with too much exaggeration.

Borderline Personality Disorder

The essential feature of this disorder is a pervasive pattern of instability of self-image, interpersonal relationships, and mood, beginning by early adulthood and present in a variety of contexts.

A marked and persistent identity disturbance is almost invariably present. This is often pervasive, and manifested by uncertainty about several life issues, such as self-image, sexual orientation, long-term goals or career choice, types of friends or lovers to have, or which values to adopt. The person often experiences this instability of self-image as chronic feelings of emptiness or boredom.

Interpersonal relationships are usually unstable and intense, and may be characterized by alternation of the extremes of over-idealization and devaluation. These people have difficulty tolerating being alone, and will make frantic efforts to avoid real or imagined abandonment.

Affective instability is common. This may be evidenced by marked mood shifts from baseline mood to depression, irritability, or anxiety, usually lasting a few hours or, only rarely, more than a few days. In addition, these people often have inappropriately intense anger or lack of control of their anger, with frequent displays of temper or recurrent physical fights. They tend to be impulsive, particularly in activities that are potentially self-damaging, such as shopping sprees, psychoactive substance abuse, reckless driving, casual sex, shoplifting and binge eating.

Recurrent suicidal threats, gestures, or behavior and other self-mutilating behavior (e.g. wrist-scratching) are common in the more severe forms of the disorder.

This behavior may serve to manipulate others, may be a result of intense anger, or may counteract feelings of "numbness" and depersonalization that arise during periods of extreme stress.

Some conceptualize this disorder as a level of personality organization rather than as a specific Personality Disorder.

Associated features. Frequently this disorder is accompanied by many features of other Personality Disorder, such as Schizotypal, Histrionic, Narcissistic and Antisocial Personality Disorders. In many cases more than one diagnosis is warranted. Quite often social contrariness and a generally pessimistic outlook are observed. Alternation between dependency and self-assertion is common. During periods of extreme stress, transient psychotic symptoms may occur, but they are generally of insufficient severity or duration to warrant an additional diagnosis.

Complications. Possible complications include Dysthymia, Major Depression, Psychoactive Substance Abuse, and psychotic disorders such as Brief Reactive Psychosis. Premature death may result from suicide.

Sex ratio. The disorder is more commonly diagnosed in females.

An example of Borderline Personality Disorder.

A certain middle-aged and ruggedly good-looking woman had a much younger and beautiful lady with her in an apartment. They were happily living together for a time. The middle-aged woman did everything for the younger lady; provided her all her needs because the middle-aged woman had a good source of income from her business shop, with the condition that the younger lady had to be faithful to her. But it was impossible for the middle-aged woman to keep all the time the younger lady away from the sight of the opposite sex. She fell in love with the guy who courted her. To make the long story short, while the middle-aged woman was out for some errands, the two secret lovers took the opportunity to leave the middle-aged woman and go to a faraway place beyond the knowledge of the latter.

The disappearance of the younger lady devastated her whole being; she had lost her wellness and beautiful outlook in life, from love to hate. She acted and behaved like a crazy woman. She vowed to kill her if she would see her with that guy, and then would kill herself.

"The fault dear Brutus is not in
the stars but in ourselves."
William Shakespeare

Avoidant Personality Disorder

The essential pattern of this disorder is a pervasive pattern of social discomfort, fear of negative evaluation, and timidity, beginning by early adulthood and present in a variety of context.

Most people somewhat concerned about how others assess them, but those with this disorder are easily hurt by criticism and are devastated by the slightest hint of disapproval. They generally are unwilling to enter into relationships unless given an unusually strong guaranteed of uncritical acceptance; consequently, they often have no close friends or confidants (or only one) other than first degree relatives.

Associated features. Depression, anxiety and anger at oneself for failing to develop social relations are commonly experienced.

Impairment. Social relations are severely restricted. Occupational functioning maybe impaired, particularly if interpersonal involvement is required.

Complications. Social phobia may be a complication of this disorder.

Predisposing factors. Avoidant disorder of Childhood or Adolescence predisposes to the development of this disorder. In addition, disfiguring physical illness may predispose to its development.

Diagnostic criteria for Avoidant Personality Disorder:

1. The person is easily hurt by criticism or disapproval.
2. The person has no close friends or confidants (or only one) other than first-degree relatives.
3. The person is unwilling to get involved with people unless certain of being liked.
4. The person avoids social or occupational activities that involve significant interpersonal contact, e.g. refuses a promotion that will increase social demands.
5. The person is reticent in social situations because of fear of saying something inappropriate or foolish, or of being unable to answer a question.
6. The person fears being embarrassed by blushing, crying, or showing signs of anxiety in front of other people.
7. The person exaggerates the potential difficulties, physical dangers or risks involved in doing something ordinary but outside his or her usual routine, e.g. may cancel social plans

because he/she anticipates being exhausted by the effort of getting there.

Management. May try long and intensive psychotherapy!

The Dependent Personality Disorder

The essential feature of this disorder is a pervasive pattern of dependent and submissive behavior beginning in early adulthood and present in a variety of contexts.

People with this disorder are unable to make everyday decisions without an excessive amount of advice and reassurance from others, and will even allow others to make most of their important decisions. For example, an adult with this disorder will typically assume a passive role and allow his or her spouse to decide where they should live, what kind of job he or she should have, and with which neighbors they should be friendly. A child or adolescent with this disorder may allow his or her parent or parents to decide what he or she should wear, with whom to associate, how to spend her free time, and what school or college to attend.

This excessive dependence on others leads to difficulty in initiating projects or doing things on one's own. People with this disorder tend to feel uncomfortable or helpless when alone, and will go to great lengths to avoid being alone. They are devastated when close relationships end, and tend to be preoccupied with fear or being abandoned.

These people are easily hurt by criticism and disapproval, and tend to subordinate themselves to others, agreeing with people even when they believe them to be wrong, for fear of being rejected. They will volunteer to do things that are unpleasant or demeaning in order to get others to like them.

Impairment. Occupational functioning maybe impaired if the job requires independence. Social relations tend to be limited to those with the few people on whom the person is dependent.

Complications. Dysthymic Disorder and Major Depression are common complications.

Diagnostic Criteria for Dependent Personality Disorder. A pervasive pattern of dependent and submissive behavior, beginning by early adulthood and present in a variety of contexts, as indicated by at least five of the following:

1. The person is unable to make everyday decisions without an excessive amount of advice or reassurance from others.
2. The person allows others to make most of his or her important decisions, e.g. where to live, what job to take.
3. The person agrees with people even when he or she believes they are wrong, because of fear or being rejected.
4. The person has difficulty initiating projects or doing things on his or her own.
5. The person volunteers to do things that are unpleasant or demeaning in order to get other people to like him or her.
6. The person feels uncomfortable or helpless when alone, or goes to great lengths to avoid being alone.
7. The person feels devastated or helpless when close relationships end.

8. The person is frequently preoccupied with fears of being abandoned.
9. The person is easily hurt by criticism or disapproval.

The Narcissistic Personality Disorder

Narcissus used to be a name of a youth in Greek Mythology. He was a good-looking youth. And he found it favorable when one day he passed by a spring and happened to see his own reflection in a spring. And because of this he was punished by the jealous gods, changing him into the flower that now bears his name, Narcissus.

Narcissistic is derived from Narcissus which means too much self-love or egocentricity. In psychoanalysis, Narcissism is the direction of a libidinal energy towards the self as the object-choice; the arrest of psycho-sexual development at the level of childish ego gratification.

The pervasive pattern of the narcissistic personality disorder of excessive emotionality and attention seeking by early adulthood and present in a variety of contexts as indicated by at least four of the following:

1. A person who seeks or demands reassurance, approval or praise.
2. A person who is not appropriately sexually seductive in appearance or behavior.
3. A person who is overly concerned with physical attractiveness.
4. A person who expresses emotion with inappropriate exaggeration, e.g., embraces casual acquaintances with excessive ardor;

uncontrollable sobbing on minor sentimental occasions, has temper tantrums.

5. A person who is uncomfortable in situations in which he or she is not the center of attention.

6. A person who displays rapidly shifting and shallow expression of emotions.

7. A person who is self-centered, actions being directed toward obtaining immediate satisfaction; has no tolerance for the frustration of delayed gratification.

8. A person who has a style of speech that is excessively impressionistic and lacking in detail, e.g., when asked to describe mother, can be no more specific than, "she was a beautiful person."

Treatment is difficult to manage in narcissistic personality disorder since it is a deeply rooted disorder in both male and female.

Obsessive-Compulsive Personality Disorder

This disorder is one of the most common personality disorder found in a competitive and highly progressive society. In fact, this particular personality type, if properly controlled, could become an ideal one. However, if it is too excessive, it will result to a pathological disorder called Neurosis. Obsessive-Compulsive Disorder is also known as Type A personality. This type of personality usually suffers from Burn-out syndrome (people who burn their candles on both ends). Many of these patients are victims of migraine, ulcers, hypertensions, heart attack, and stroke.

Diagnostic and Statistical Manual III (DSM-111) defines obsessive-compulsive disorder as a pervasive pattern of perfectionism and inflexibility that starts in early adolescence.

Here are the characteristic traits of the Obsessive-Compulsive Personality Disorder: (A Summary)

1. He is a stubborn person.
2. He worries constantly.
3. He cannot relax.
4. He is insecure.
5. He is an over sensitive person; he cannot tolerate criticism, but he is critical of others.
6. He adheres to strict rules as a way of covering his insecurity.
7. He refuses to assume blame for his mistakes.
8. He wants to be perfect all the time.
9. He is stingy with money, love and time.
10. Secretly, he often questions his own salvation.

Obsessive-Compulsive Personality Disorder is common among males. It is genetically endowed.

Treatment: Quite difficult to treat. Spiritual therapy might help.

Bipolar Affective Disorder

Psychiatrists have been treating a fairly good number of Filipinos who are sick with this particular **mood disorder** in contrast distinction with schizophrenia which is **mental disorder.** Studies have shown that one of the major causes of this disorder is the deep-seated unresolved conflict between the hostile mother and the vindictive daughter who becomes hyperactive when one breaks down.

Bipolar affective disorder is a long-term recurrent

mood disorder characterized by the presence of both depressive and manic phases and moods.

The depressive changes could be manifested by irritability, loss of interest or pleasure in all activities, loss of appetite, sleep energy, and concentration; feeling of worthlessness, excessive guilt; recurrent thoughts of death or suicidal attempts. The manic phase or mood disorder is manifested by inflated self-esteem or grandiosity ("I am the brightest"), more talkative than usual; flight of ideas or thoughts are racing; easy distractibility, excessive involvement in pleasurable activities; the patient is mentally and physically hyperactive than usual. These symptoms may continue for more than two weeks. The patient's social and occupational activities are impaired most victims are described to be above average in intelligence.

Patients suffering from this disorder are considered high risks to themselves and others. Hence, they need to be confined in an isolation cell for proper management and for security. Today, there are effective medications for bipolar affective disorder but their doses should be properly monitored by laboratory procedures. Psychotherapy is also a must to prevent early recurrence.

Mania-A Common Mood Disorder

Conventionally, in Mania, the patient is said to be suffering from Bipolar Disorder (DMS-III) or Manic Depressive Disorder.

Mania is also synonymously known as effective, mood or emotional disorder. Candidates to this illness are mostly women with higher I.Q. than normal. Manic patients are easier to treat than Schizophrenic patients because they respond better to antipsychotic medications. It has a strong genetic predisposition.

There are many Filipinos who are victims or ill with this affective or emotional illness taking into account that we are a very highly emotional people. Hence, in my professional practice, I have treated a lot of manic patients. Incidentally, mood disorder is not the classical Mental Disorder like the Schizophrenic Disorder whose characteristic behavior is totally shattered and extremely bizarre. Manic Disorder is relatively easier to treat than Schizophrenic Disorder.

The Classical Symptoms of Manic Disorder:

1. A distinct period of abnormally and persistently elevated, expansive, or extremely irritable mood.
2. Inflated self-esteem or grandiosity (I am the best...).
3. Decrease need for sleep or inability to sleep.
4. More talkative than usual or pressure to keep talking on any topic (with coherence).
5. Easily distractive and talks in irrelevant topics he/she is easily drawn to.
6. Increase in goal-directed activity, like interest in work, business, socials, school, sexual or psychomotor agitation. They act on them, they are unrestrained.
7. They are high risk to commit violence, and may commit suicide.
8. They are all hyperactive physically, mentally and emotionally.
9. Speech is loud, rapid and hard to understand and to interrupt.
10. They manifest flight of ideas–– a continuous uninterrupted speech from one topic to another.

Management:

Refer to a Psychiatrist for proper handling. Hospitalization is needed and effective antipsychotic medication is indicated.

Generalized Anxiety Disorder

A fairly good number of male and female Filipinos at the ages of 20 and 30 years are referred for psychiatric treatment for their frequent complaint of severe anxiety (grabing *kulba*). These individuals are known as *"nerbyoso or tarantado kayo* in the local dialect. All these victims are not aware of the causes of their feelings.

This behavioral change of anxiety and tension could be traced back to a childhood trauma when the child was constantly exposed to severe experiences of fear such as loud sounds. Examples: Frightening thunder, shouting, treats of near death or annihilation, evil spirits, other fearful stories of ghosts, etc. that conditioned the child to a state of vulnerability, helplessness and fearfulness.

The essential feature of this disorder is unrealistic or excessive anxiety and worry (apprehensive expectation) about two or more like circumstances, e.g., worry about possible misfortune to one's child (who is in no danger) and worry about finances (for no good reason), for six months or longer, during which the person has been bothered by these concerns more days than not. In children and adolescents this may take the form of anxiety and worry about academic, athletic, and social performance.

Symptoms of Generalized Anxiety Disorder:

1. Symptoms of motor tension include trembling, twitching or feeling shaky; muscle tension and aches or soreness; restlessness; easy fatigability.
2. Symptoms of automatic hyperactivity include: Shortness of breath or smothering sensations; palpitations or accelerated heart rate (tachycardia); sweating, or cold clammy hands; dry mouth; dizziness or lightheadedness; nausea, diarrhea, or other abnormal distress; flushes (hot flushes) or chills; frequent urination; and trouble swallowing or a "lump in the throat".
3. Symptoms of vigilance and scanning include: feeling keyed up or on edge; exaggerated startle and response, difficulty concentrating or mind going blank because of anxiety; trouble falling or staying asleep; and irritability.

Management:

An intensive psychotherapy is indicated with the aid of anti-anxiety agents to help them become well!

Birth Order Influences One's Personality

Several studies made by top psychologist abroad claim that the position you are in the Birth Order influences more than your childhood experiences. It shapes your adult personality. Birth order traits are distinct and predictable. Behaviorists have summed up the impact of Birth order in the following characteristic traits profile:

- **The Firstborn Child.** Oldest children are described to be serious, hardworking and high achievers. Why? Because they strive for adult approval. They are also conformists who would follow the rules. They tend to be straight forward in their dealings with others. Oldest children are more apt to reach the top of their profession. They do better in school. Survey states that a high percentage of honor students are oldest children. There are more gifted children and men of science among the firstborn than later-born. They are also likely to be more dependent, conservative and suggestible.
- **The Middle Child.** Second-born children are known as "social siblings." They are described to be easy-going, cheerful and charming. They may be rebellious within the family, but outside, they are conformists and they are usually very popular with their peers. They are less aggressive and may apt-out of competition with more powerful older siblings.
- **The Youngest Child.** Youngest siblings are often strongly influenced by older brothers and sisters. They tend to be idealistic, creative, and subject to moodiness. They are often spoiled and overprotected. Because they are constantly striving to catch up with elder siblings, most develop an "I'll show you" attitude and may take on huge workload to gain acceptance. According to Alfred Adler they continue to expect attention and "fight for a place in the sun" and develop a competitive spirit.
- **The Only Child.** Only children are said to be

more confident and less competitive than other kids. They are relaxed about life and assume that they can get what they want without much trouble. They tend to be pampered and longed to have another sibling as his/her constant companion.

Of course, there are still other significant factors that can contribute to mold one's personality make-up: genetic, ambition, education, experience, diligence, consistency, opportunity, perseverance, and a strong spiritual program.

"Distorted Thinking" Most People Commit

"A man who has committed mistakes
and does not make effort to correct them
will continue to do the same mistakes."
Anonymous

One of the most effective methods of psychotherapy that psychotherapists use in their counseling is **"Cognitive Therapy"** as advocated by doctors A. beck and D. Burns. These common self-defeating thought patterns which are known as "inner-saboteurs" (Destructive thoughts) are the sources of man's negative feelings of anxiety depression and psychosomatic disorders.

Let us mention some examples of these adverse **distorted thoughts:**

1. <u>Jumping to conclusion</u>. People who use this thinking as if they "read minds" without validating their assumptions. They judge right away based on their bias attitude,

2. <u>All of nothing thinking</u>. A person who sees everything in black and white. A student who gets one B and thinks he is a total failure.
3. <u>Overgeneralization</u>. A person who expects and concludes a uniform of bad luck because of one bad experience.
4. <u>Mental filtering.</u> One who sees a negative fragment of a situation and dwells on it. He soon concludes that everything is negative.
5. <u>Automatic discounting.</u> The way one who often brushes aside a compliment. He concludes right away that "he is just being nice." But he does not believe it for he thinks it's insincere.
6. <u>Magnification and minimization.</u> This is like a "binocular trick" because one either blows things up or shrinks them out of proportion. As if one is always looking at his imperfection and everything through a binocular.
7. <u>Emotional reasoning</u>. A person says "I feel guilty: therefore I must have done something bad." A projection of a negative thought.
8. Should statements. People say, "I should do this" or "I must do that," a thinking of most blind and unreasonable people who want to show dominance-right or wrong, no exceptions, as they have learned from their parents or teachers.
9. Labeling and mislabeling. There are persons who think, "I'm a failure" instead of "I made a mistake." Such labeling is irrational.
10. <u>Personalization</u>. A person who thinks whatever happens, whatever others do, it's his fault. Dr. Burns says, "You suffer from a paralyzing sense of bogus guilt." What another person does is

ultimately his or her responsibility, not yours. There are still many other distorted thinking.

Here are realistic thinking to replace negative thoughts:

- Your feelings are not facts.
- You can cope up with the real problems and will come less painful.
- Don't base your opinion of yourself on your achievements. You can't base your self-worth on looks, talents, fame or fortune. Only your own true sense of self-worth determines how you feel. Be your humble self, always be honest and sincere. God knows you well, man. Change your negative attitudes. Okay?

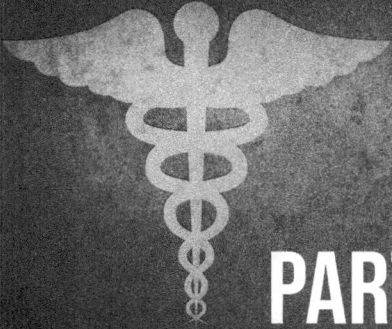

PART V

"HOW TOS" FOR PERSONAL IMPROVEMENT

The Art of Changing Oneself

Of all the creatures that God the Father has created to have dominion over the rest of His created things in this planet Earth is Man.

Man was created after God's own likeness, with body and soul and is endowed with the highest intelligence, so much so that man could easily adjust and change his way of life to improve the pattern of his own lifestyle.

The sages say: "Man is the architect of his own destiny." To the Greeks: "Man's fate is the result of his action." The famous American Psychologist, William James, declared that the greatest revolution in his generation was the discovery that human beings, by changing the inner attitudes of their minds, can change the outer aspects of their lives.

History and literature are full of inspirational examples of the miracle of inner change. Do you know the Persian story of the hunchback prince who became straight and tall by standing each day before a statue of himself made straight?

- Real change requires the substituting of new habits for the old ones. Mold your character and future by your thoughts and acts.
- Change can be advanced by associating with men whom you could walk among the stars.
- Change can be inspired by selecting your own spiritual ancestors from among the great of all ages. You can practice the kindliness of Lincoln, the devotion of Schweitzer, the vision of Franklin.
- Change can be achieved by changing your environment. Let go of the lower things and reach for the higher. Surround yourself with the best in books, music and art.
- Change can be accomplished most of all through the power of prayers, because with God all things are possible.

How to Improve Your Memory

*"When one is right, no one remembers;
when one is wrong, no one forgets."*
Irish Proverb

Memory is so essential function to man. It is the power to recall or remember the past. How much we appreciate people who have a very retentive memory! How embarrassing it is for one not to remember the name of a close friend whom he has been associated with since childhood. And how pitiful it is for a young student who has been long in school because he could hardly pass in almost all his subjects due to poor memory!

Authorities say that our memory is like any muscle-the more it is exercised, the stronger it gets. Here are some time-proven techniques to improve your memory.

- Intend to remember and concentrate very well. Remembering is largely a matter of motivation-you have to want to remember.
- Understand well what you are trying to remember. Vague or illogical things are hard or difficult to remember.
- Organize well what you know into an important pattern. It's easier to find what you want in a well-kept filling cabinet.
- Become interested in what you want to remember. An avid basketball fan has no trouble remembering his favorite players shooting average.
- The law of Association. Associating an idea with another idea; or a thing or object with another thing or object.
- Use as many senses as possible. Repeating a name aloud, when you are introduced to someone involves sight, small writing cards, etc. (descriptive memory).
- The best time to memorize is before bedtime and immediately after rising. In this way, your mind and subconscious mind are still undisturbed.
- Lot of worries or unresolved personal conflicts will obstruct good memory function.
- Pray to the Holy Spirit for good memory retention.

How to Beat Loneliness

Everyone must have experienced the pangs of being lonely in this life. When God created Adam in the Garden of Eden, God realized that Adam was so alone and it was not good for man to be lonely, he should have a loving companion. So God created Eve by plucking a rib from Adam's side and lo, Eve evolved.

We Filipinos are known to be a sentimental people. When a loved one goes away to work abroad, or even just to take a long vacation, people who are left behind would easily cry, and would feel very lonely. They would lose their appetite and could not sleep at night. This feeling of depression would go several days and nights. Many of these weak-willed people would even get sick and become so thin and emaciated and some may land in the psychiatric ward.

Authorities suggest some measures to conquer loneliness.

- Well, have a good cry. It is therapeutic to pour your tears as a check-valve during sudden departures.
- Be good to yourself. Seek the company of your friends and have a good time. Enjoy and beat the blues.
- Realize that you are not alone.
- Break the bad habit of isolating yourself.
- Act like an enthusiastic person.
- Associate with enthusiastic people.
- Practice hope until you can achieve a happy spirit.

- Seek a credible counselor to help you resolve your serious problems in life.
- Always pray to God to help you live a Christ-centered life!

How to Conquer Frustrations

From birth to death, people are experiencing failures that make them feel frustrated!

Here are some common experiences of human frustrations. There are couples who could not bear any child at all, despite specialist's help. There are graduate professionals who have been taking the Board or Bar Examination several times. There are promising and ambitious politicians but unfortunately died in a plane crush. And so many victims of natural disasters, etc., some parents have children who were born blind, retarded, etc.

Psychologists and other authorities suggest positive ways on how to combat frustrations:

1. Resign to the will of God. Probably God gives you this trial as your Way to Heaven, that is if you accept it without complaining.
2. Don't indulge in self-pity. Positively think that it's your bad day and also think that there still many good days to come. Here is an inspiring saying, "If Winter comes, can spring be far behind?"
3. Always foster positive thinking.
4. Cultivate the virtue of optimism.
5. Don't be easily discouraged.
6. Plan and study well your moves and remember always the saying, "Look before you leap."

7. If venturing on a project be sure you have enough resources to sustain you.
8. Have an indomitable patience.
9. Learn muscular relaxation technique.
10. Before you sleep flush out of your mind all negative thoughts.
11. Rely on Almighty God's guidance.

How to Achieve Your Physical Well-being

Recently, in a birthday party attended by some relatives and close friends, I met a long lost friend who came from the U.S. We used to play "Tarzan-Tarzan" together in their fruit farm in Valencia, Negros Oriental, during summer vacation. Both of us were enthusiasts in health and body building, inspired by the famous culturist like Charles Atlas with his dynamic tension system and who earned the title of "the most perfectly developed body." And I also showed him the U.S. Strength and Health Magazine that I had. He used to lend me some of his series of Tarzan Books by Edgar R. Burroughs. It was really fun when we used to compare our gains in chest and other muscle bulk measurements.

Well, that was our adolescent history in the making! But years passed, he must be in his late 70's now. I can't believe it, his physique is still looking terrific! I asked him his secret. Well, he is still maintaining a regular program of exercise, high protein diet, etc. to keep him fit and strong.

The following are his routine program:

• Eat nourishing foods: fresh milk, fruit and vegie drinks, etc. Stay away from fatty foods. Boil, bake, or grill. Never fry.

- Take prescribe supplements.
- Don't eat when you are upset (angry). Uncontrolled hostility at meal time turns food sour and brings ulcers and heart problems, studies show.
- Tension and worry bring physical and emotional illness (stress). Get your mind off your work. A good medical advice–– "placidity prevents acidity."
- Exercise is a must. Do regular aerobics–– walking, swimming, etc.
- Rest and relaxation are important, too. Recreate with your family. Take a vacation.
- Loss of energy is due to boredom. Take on challenges, new interest. Enjoy life.
- Conserve energy. Give in a little at times. Apply discipline and do every job with love and enthusiasm.
- Avoid stress and heavy strain. Take charge of your mind and your mind will take charge of your body.
- See your doctor for any complaint...and always thank God for a healthy well-being!

How to Keep on Living and not just Existing

Philosophers can well differentiate between living and existing. They can tell if a person has lived to the fullest or if a person just merely exists without any focus or not knowing its purpose of his existence.

Many of us observed that a person who is really alive is bubbling with vim, vigor and vitality. He is always on the go and is sensitive to the people around him. To him, looking good is feeling good inside. In any activity, he does his best and always dreaming big. He never forget to say "Thanks" when God answers his prayers.

The following are some admirable traits of an active person in the society.

- He likes people.
- He is a sociable person.
- He has many interests in life; friends, books, music, art, travel, etc.
- He realizes that sorrows and trouble are part of life that he can overcome through prayers and sacrifices.
- He always lives in the present.
- He believes that interest is the measure of aliveness,
- To him, to know God is to live.

How to Beat the Stress of Worrying

Here is a good reminder by Robert Frost on the problem of worry: "The reason why worry kills more people than work is that more people indulge in worry than work." This truism is also applied by another American writer, Beecher, who said: "Work does not kill man, it is worry. Work is healthy. You can hardly put on man that he cannot bear. Worry is rust upon the blade. It's not the revolution that destroys the machinery but the friction."

We were told in Genesis that when God created Adam and Eve, He provided them with their basic needs in the Garden of Eden. However, when they transgressed God's commandment, then, they were punished...they and their children and all their descendants started to feel the problems of life. Hence, they have now to worry in order to survive, and live from the "sweat of their brows!"

Today, Filipinos have been beset with the changes of modern life and many have adopted the Western lifestyle-from fashion, food, entertainment, etc. the consequences are enormous. Many have been victimized by the "future shock" of the American ways of life. Many Filipinos have become "neurotic"-a condition of the mind that would make the person react and negatively magnifies a slight or even a harmless thing to a level of high anxiety, thus making a person extremely worried. If this troublesome anxiety is not treated, the person may suffer depression that may lead to suicide or possibly a psychosis or mental breakdown. Hence, the statement: "Worry kills."

Here are steps to manage the stress of worrying:

- Always be realistic. We have to admit the truth that what we have "to fear most is fear itself." (F. Roosevelt.) Most successful people say that there are no obstacles in life, only challenges.
- Treat worries and problems as opportunistic challenges which require immediate action. A fresh renewed approach often creates wonders!
- If you are warned by the pressure of any problem that is worrying you, you have to take instant action to avert real trouble. Don't just ignore it for worry doesn't easily go away.
- Seek out a close friend with whom you can discuss your problem. A good deal of tension can be relieved by talking your trouble over with an uninvolved and trusted friend.
- Don't blame your problems on others. It helps to remember that nobody is always right. If

you are wrong, admit it. It's the only way to avert ugly quarrels.

- All work and no play make Jack a dull boy. Take out for fun, hobbies, ballgames, or any form of leisure and relaxation. This will unwind your nerves.
- Always pray to the Almighty God "to listen your heavy load and He will give you rest!"

Boredom

*"When there ceases to be a
sense of newness, challenge and
excitement, we all get bored."*
Susan Heitler

There are people who get easily bored. They live with routine activities and doing the same monotonous work pattern day-in and day-out. These humdrum activities could drive one to boredom.

To most people, boredom would simply mean monotony, dullness, apathy, tediousness, wearisome, ennui, and languor. Hence, the expression-"I am bored to death!"

Authorities say that our mind needs a steady diet of new input, the same way that our body needs fresh and nourishing food, otherwise, we feel bored or stressed. Boredom can be psychologically become very painful for it contributes to depression or erode our self-esteem. However, psychologists say that boredom is curable.

Here are some remedial suggestions to rid boredom:

1. Don't be tense-relax. When you are bored, your tendency is to get away (escape to laziness)

from what bores you. But you are unable to do this because you feel guilty (you are forced to do your work). So, you become tense. But the routine vicious process make the reluctant person become too apathetic, bored, lethargic, too tired and sleepy.

2. Take a break from your routine work. For instance, go out (instead of studying in the boarding house, go to the library and study there instead); or you may eat out in some affordable eatery together with some friends, etc.

3. Set aside a day and see a nice movie; window shopping; play badminton or any indoor game to maintain health. Vary your activities.

4. Keep in touch and expand your circle of friends. Everybody needs human contact. Text some people who can uplift your mood. Chat with them and invite them to go out with you.

5. Go to a bookstore and buy some interesting piece of literature; buy a joke pocket book, etc.

6. Listen to lively music to make your mind alert and spirited. Avoid mournful or sentimental type of music that depresses you.

7. Do yourself a "private hour" each day. Redo your hair; polish or color your nails; read hilarious books; make a profitable hobby, etc.

8. Devise ways and means to do your work better-this is "creativity." And always discover something new, something that challenges you or give a sense of decent excitement.

Try always to see the sunny side of life. Learn to laugh at yourself and the incongruities of life to remain sane and put an end to boredom. God wants us to be peaceful and happy people and never to be bored.

Character

> *"When wealth is lost, nothing is lost.*
> *When health is lost, something is lost.*
> *When character is lost, all is lost."*
>
> Anonymous

Question: Why has Christ become a very well-known person during his time? Answer: Because he was doing good all the time. In this world, the good as well as the bad persons co-exist like the weeds and good plants growing together in the same garden. To the anthropologist a man is composed of good and bad elements depending on the prevailing circumstance of either positive or negative factors that trigger the reaction.

Someone fittingly describes man as a creature who makes the desert bloom and the lake die. Connoting that man is a *"builder* and a *destroyer"* at the same time.

Let me cite the good behavior of man-his *character* traits. Character is the dominant quality of a person's traits, temperament, mood, attitude and nature. An American writer, Steven R. Covey, says that character is made up of the principles and values that give one's life direction, meaning and depth. These constitute one's inner sense of what is right and wrong based not on laws or rules of conduct but on *what he is*. Basically, character includes admirable traits such as *integrity, honesty, courage, fairness, helpfulness, cheerfulness, generosity, loyalty, religiosity, etc.*

It is a common human nature that a man never

discloses his own character as clearly as when he describes another. People always become so perceptive when it comes to assessing the character faults of others but always minimizing their own character faults. The things he loathed in others as anger and resentment existed in him. Psychologists call this as "projection (ascribing one's own weakness to others-a common defense mechanism).

Honorable men say that character are in the dark (Dwight Mood). The happiness of every country depends on the character of the people, rather than the form of government it has (Thomas Holeburton).

Definitely, we can *only* experience true success, peace and happiness in the world by making character the bedrock and paradigm of our lives.

Controversial Maturity

*"Those trees that are slow to
grow, bear the best fruits."*

Moliere

Maturity is a controversial word. For when a person reaches adulthood, age 20 and above, he said to be "mature," but probably in his chronological age *only* as he appears physically. However, his behavior, especially his emotion, shows that he is still immature or childish in many ways-egocentric, impulsive, irresponsible and oversensitive. Immature behavior is a common major cause of marital rifts or unwanted marriages as well as personality defects.

Let us then analyze what true maturity is. Authorities basically define maturity as the full <u>development of man's physical and mental attributes</u>. It is the state of being truly mature and the realization of the full potentiality for human development–– the height of maturation process.

Here are some important criteria for being a mature person:

- A person is said to be mature if he has the ability to control adequately his emotions like anger or temper, and settle his differences without resorting to violence or destruction.
- Maturity is well manifested by patience, the willingness to postpone immediate pleasure. The immature person always say, "I want NOW!"
- The individual who keeps changing his jobs, friends and marriage partners is immature.
- The mature person could resign to the shortcomings in life, accepts defeat and constructive criticism.
- Maturity means loyalty to one's good legal spouse, friends and employers.
- Maturity is the ability to live up to one's responsibilities and keeping one's word or promise.
- Maturity is the capacity to face unpleasantness and disappointments without rancor or becoming bitter.
- Maturity is the ability to make decisions. An immature person can't decide on serious matters, but depends mostly on others (wife, mother, friends) to make the decision for him.
- Maturity is unselfishness responding to the needs of others.
- Maturity is humility. A mature person is able to

say, "I was wrong," or "I am sorry." And when he is proved rights, he does not say, "I told you so."
- Maturity means discipline, dependability, flexibility, integrity and diligence. The immature person has excuses for everything. He blames the whole world for his failures.
- And finally, maturity is the capacity to live in peace with that which he cannot change. He is a true instrument of good service.

Eric Berne says, "A real mature person must know how to blend and integrate his three ego states–– he should know when he is behaving as a good PARENT, a responsible ADULT and a fun-loving CHILD.

The Challenge of Breaking Bad Habits

Some bad habits are so firmly rooted in our lives so much so that they seem impossible to be conquered. Probably many of us have seen people who become so fat or obese that they look like Japanese sumo wrestlers. Once they would decide to reduce, they usually group together and pledge to follow a very strict program of very rigid exercises that would make them sweat so much until those fats are melted. This process of making them thin takes several months or even years.

The problem with a recalcitrant habit is that it can produce a deep sense of frustration. A lot of weak-willed people have given up the hard struggle and would die with their destructive habits because of hopelessness and worthlessness.

Psychologists have devised effective steps in behavioral change.

1. DESIRE. If you really want to change a bad behavior then you must make a strong positive effort to do it all "though hell should bar the way!"
2. KNOWLEDGE. One must learn all the secrets of how to overcome this destructive habit.
3. VISUALIZATION. You should see the positive gains of your efforts
4. PLANNING. Be sure to follow all the effective steps. Remember: "No pain, no gain."
5. ACTION. Do it! There are no excuses. Show to the world how you win the hardest battle in your life.

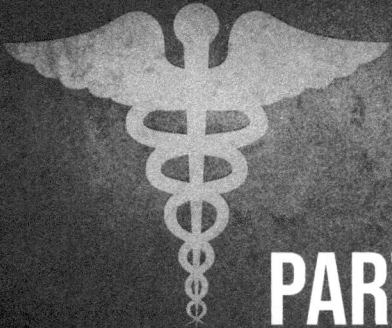

PART VI

IMPORTANT THINGS TO KNOW FOR HUMAN GROWTH AND DEVELOPMENT

The Importance of Knowing Our Roots

One area in our life we seem to take for granted is our past, especially our family history. We should try to assemble all the puzzle pieces of our past so that we could come to a better understanding of ourselves; who we are, why we behave, think and feel as we do, and where we are going. We cannot fully understand ourselves if we do not know our family history, our heritage, and our roots or origin of our humble beginning.

Counseling and psychotherapy, if they are given any value, must deal with client's roots. It was the famous historian, George Santayana, who said, "If one does not know his past, he is bound to repeat it." This means that we should all know the major pitfalls, the causes of our failures, the hereditary tendencies; our talents and capabilities our Creator has given us in this life. The good and beneficial tendencies must be developed properly and live well in order to be successful and be happy in this life. The human weakness–– vices and bad habits should be avoided at all costs.

Unfortunately, some people were born poor, homeless and jobless. But through sheer faith, strivings, and hard work, they emerged successfully in their undertakings.

A person who knows how to cultivate and nourish his roots will always be rewarded by God. For instance, a person who experiences extreme deprivation in life due to the early death of his parents, in order to survive, he helps in his uncle's Duck Farm. In so doing, accompanied with patience and perseverance he is able to support his studies until college, specializing in Agri-Business. Through hard work, he is able to establish his own Balut (cooked fertilized egg) Factory. He receives orders here and there, making him richer and richer every day. He is now known as the Silent Millionaire in Luzon. Every time he is invited to talk in some gatherings, he never fails to mention about his roots and humble beginnings and acknowledges that all blessings come from God!

The Importance of Good Relationships

The expression-"No man is an island but part of the main," clearly emphasizes the fact that nobody in this wide world can survive if he lives alone in utter isolation. When God created Paradise, He also created Adam. But he said, "Man should not be alone." So, He created Eve to be Adam's companion. This is the start of human social relationship. Then, the first parents formed the first family, until they multiply and peopled the earth.

Studies show the great importance of good relationships-families, relatives and friends who live harmoniously and peacefully–– live much longer as compared to those whose social relationships or connections are few or absent. Even people who tend to plants and pets live longer than a solitary soul. Relationships are so essential to a long and healthy life.

Sometimes we are alone by choice or by some circumstances. But there's a big difference between being alone and being lonely. For instance, some people live alone and have few friends, but they fill their lives with wholesome activities and interests. This is not so bad. Why? They are happy, contented and feel fulfilled. They aren't lonely. Other people can be lonely in a room full of families and acquaintances. For some reasons, they don't make personal connections well. They shun socialization. By nature they are loners. These people can feel isolated even if they are around people all the time.

Sociologists and psychologists report that people who regularly give and receive affection are much healthier in general, live, longer and enjoy a higher quality of life than those who do not. Here's a great saying, "The key is to love and be loved." It's an important part of the overall balance and lifestyle in one's life.

Here are some tips for bringing sound relationships in one's life:

- Be sure to make time for friends. A social network of friends help fights loneliness and isolation. It prevents depression, anxiety, boredom, dissatisfied feelings and poor health. A company of faithful friends can help one achieve good feelings and positive emotions.
- Get out and socialize. Don't be an isolationist. When friends call to invite you out with them, don't decline. Accept the invitation.
- Stay in touch with your close relatives. As we grow older, we miss a lot of trusted relatives. They may migrate to far places or may have

already died. You may greet or Email them regularly, eat out with them, see a movie, or picnicking with them, etc.

- Now is the time to mend broken relationships, too. Remember that life is too short to harbor grudges, or mourn lost relationships. By all means, before you say goodbye to this world, be sure to settle and put aside your differences. As St. Francis of Assisi said, "It is in forgiving that we are forgiven."

So, don't fear relationships! Share what you have with your friends-your nearest neighbor." This is a true sign of maturity and a self-fulfillment!

The Importance of Right Motivation

In this modem world, people usually ask the secret of men who become successful and those who suffer from utter failure. Authorities who scientifically studied claim the important factor behind success or failure of any career. In this modem world, people usually ask the secret of men who become successful and those who in life which is **motivation.**

The dictionary of psychology defines **motivation** as the incentive (both intrinsic and extrinsic) which initiates and sustains any given activity. It is a goal directed behavior. In this definition, it is clear that people who like to do righteous things are truly motivated. But individuals who refuse to do a given task is not properly motivated. Don't waste your time and energy on them. People who accept work or job where they are not trained or qualified will never prosper but sure to fail. They are said to be "Square pegs in round holes."

There was once a Medical Director of a hospital who strongly motivated his brilliant son to take up medicine. The obedient son followed his over ambitious father to become a doctor, though his magnificent obsession was to become a priest, as motivated by his loving mother and the chaplain of the school where he studied.

One day, he came to realize that he could not become a "Servant of the Lord." He suffered mental anguish and uttered frustration...he lost his sanity. He was preaching Gospels at the hospital ground of his father. The late Msgr. Tudtud said, "He could have been a brilliant prelate."

There were those promising professionals whose career were good, however many of them were motivated by big monetary gains, so much so that they became corrupt and materialistic. And still they wanted to run for high ranking positions in the government.

The best motivation is follow Jesus Christ who said, "I am the Way, the Truth, and the Life."

The Importance of Common Sense

When I was young, my Dad, who used to be a Biology teacher at the Negros Oriental High School had taught me and my other siblings a lot of beneficial lessons on how to be a good, knowledgeable person not only about things we basically learned in school, but most importantly on things that would make us use our common sense to make us good, wise, most practical and gentle people. To my dad, a real man is one who knows how to be responsible, independent and flexible and can do a lot of common sense.

We cannot deny that in this world people differ in talents. And let us remember the moral lesson we learned from the short story (fable) of the mountain and the squirrel. "You can carry a forest at your back but neither can you crack a nut!"

We are living in very challenging words of common sense! There are people who are so dogmatic and so absolute and exacting in their words as if they are perfect. Example: "Dark cloud always brings rain." The truth is: "dark cloud does not always bring rain."

Here are some reflections of common sense that are true to life:

- A mole can teach a philosopher on the art of digging a hole.
- The one who is not hungry calls the coconut shells hard.
- The bullfrog knows better about rain than the almanac.
- "One pound of learning requires 10 pounds of common sense to apply it (Persian proverb).
- One hand cannot tie a bundle.
- (An equalizer)-Black cow also gives white milk.
- Dirty water will also wash dirt.
- Every family has a skeleton in the closet.
- If one has common sense, he can talk to cattle (Swiss proverb).

Why can people of good nature talk and understand the nature (behavior) of plants and animals? Saints claim that even living plants and animals have sentient souls! Hence, they can also feel like human beings. They bleed when they are pricked...they also need tender and loving care, like us. These living creatures essentially need our common sense to let them grow and propagate. If we neglect their basic needs, they will die!

"If you wish to be blamed, marry! But if you wish to be praised, die! For heaven's sake, use your common sense!"

The Importance of Hugging

Hugging is a common approved non-verbal way of greetings in a peaceful and well-bred society.

Different cultures have their own way of greeting and showing their utmost respect even with strangers. The Eskimos rub their noses; the Russians hug (bear bug) and kiss the checks; but majority just extend their hands for a handshake. But Filipinos imitate the Western style-hug and touch check-to-check.

Studies by both psychologists and social scientists claim that hugging is a very vital major healing activity. It has been proven that hugging is an important sense of touch that makes people feel good. Infants left in a crib without human contact are easily vulnerable to suffer from illnesses and die.

Surprisingly and ironically, there are still some individuals in our society who frown upon hugging. These are the bigoted people who were raised in an extremely malicious and moralistic family atmosphere. They project hugging as a highly sexualized behavior or an immoral act. They have a bad conscience. Please avoid them.

Health authorities always advice to hug every friend or relative you meet and let yourself by hugged by them. Hugging is a priceless gift or gesture you, as a true Christian, can give a weary soul.

The Importance of Punctuality

Undeniably, one of the most unbecoming cultural traits of many of our brother Filipinos is habitual unfaithfulness to their appointments. This is really shameful behavior but people just commonly ignore it and many will rationalize it as "Filipino time." No, Sir! It is high time to cut this bad trait especially now that a lot of foreign nationals are not only visiting us but living with us.

Why does punctuality matter? Sociologists have found that arriving at appointments at bit ahead of time actually reduces stress. Punctuality also enhances a person's reputation. Henry Adams says, "Punctuality preserves peace and good temper in a family or business. It gives calmness of mind. It gives insight to character. It is contagious and thus leads to a general saving of time, temper, and money."

Punctuality indicates competence. When one is on time, it shows that he tries to be in-control of his life, instead of allowing any circumstance to prevent him from doing the things he wants to do.

Punctuality suggests dependability. In society where promises are often broken and commitments frequently ignored, people appreciate those who stick to their word. Dependable people earn the respect from friends and family. Employers value those who arrive on time for work and meet deadlines. Dependable workers may even be rewarded with a higher salary and greater trust and respect.

What can one do to be punctual? Here are some practical ways to do:

1. If you find that you are regularly late for appointments, perhaps your schedule is too full. Why not cut none essential time wasters?

There are people who are too meticulous and waste too much time talking and explaining things in an overly detailed manner which is not necessary.

2. Schedule more time between appointments and aim to arrive early. This will allow for unexpected circumstances such as traffic congestion or bad weather condition.

3. You should also know your limitations. Decide whether an appointment or deadline will realistically fit your schedule before agreeing to it.

4. Avoid overbooking or receiving too many schedules for this will definitely add stress and frustrations to oneself and to others.

5. The Holy Bible tells us to make the best use of our time (Ephesians 5:15, 16).

The Importance of Self-Esteem

In this world, it is very important to know yourself. Philosophers would essentially say, "Know thyself." This basically means that every man worth his salt, should know his innate strengths i.e. talents, capabilities, goals, etc. as well as his weaknesses i.e. fears, bad habits, negative attitudes, etc. to be able to move on and have a better outlook in life.

Let us first define what self-esteem means. Self-Esteem refers to the self-evaluation of our worth, competence and importance as a person. Self-esteem basically includes our thoughts, feelings, emotions, desires, values, attitudes toward ourselves. Positive self-esteem is a healthy personal condition which practices contentment and self-worth. Whereas, impaired or negative self-esteem is an unhealthy condition which produces a sense of inferiority, inadequacy which may eventually lead to a feeling of depression.

Let me cite an example. I know of a young female, a college graduate from a known university who passed the board examination with a high rating. This girl suffered from a recurrent depression without the benefit of any therapy. She belonged to an average family of five siblings with four girls and one boy. This pretty girl even became chosen as the town's May Flower Queen during her late childhood. Her nagging complaint was-"I am an ugly duckling," she being *kayumangi* (slightly darker skin complexion). She was so distraught about her skin. One day, she became so despondent that she committed suicide. This is what a very poor self-esteem can do to an emotionally unstable person.

Studies show that the most effective therapy in a person with self-esteem is what we call as "Cognitive Behavior Therapy (CBT). The therapist can help the subject by teaching him to understand and correct his irrational thought patterns and replacing them with positive though processes. This is what Rev. Norman V. Peale underwent in conquering his very poor self-esteem. Remember: "We are all children of God" (Ephesus 2:10). Nobody can deprive us of this prime privilege and honor.

The Importance of Communication

*"When you have nothing
to say, say nothing."*
Charles Colton

We are now living the Age of Communication. The

20th century witnessed a communication revolution primarily in terms of increased telecommunication inventions, access and networking. However, I would like to emphasize only on personal communication.

Talking is the most common way of human communication. Verbal communication means using words to express thoughts, ideas, beliefs and wants. Your manner of talking and what you say will also reflect the kind of character you have as a person. Although there are exceptions.

Studies have shown that one of the major causes of impaired interpersonal relationships is due to poor communication between people. For instance, as an Expert Witness is marital court cases, I had been attesting to the fact that one of the major issues in marital rifts is usually due to innuendoes, insults, and nasty words coming from the mouth or wife which happen most especially when their ego is hurt. Some may apologize and ask for forgiveness later for what they have uttered, but the emotional wound had already been inflicted and the scar remains. So, it is important to be careful when you talk to prevent misunderstandings and quarrels.

Remember this Biblical passage: "A soft answer, turns away wrath." (Proverbs 15:1NKJV) I want to share a practical report from "Teen Health" book on good communication which is essentially based on two parts, namely: (a) speaking skills, and (b) listening skills. Here are some useful guides.

Speaking skills:

- Think before you speak to avoid embarrassment or misunderstanding.
- Avoid nonstop talking.

- Be direct and say only what is important.
- Be positive. (Be enthusiastic when you talk.)
- Be simple and talk clearly so as not to confuse your listener.
- Otherwise, you may just print or write your message to have less mistakes.

Listening skills:

This requires "active listening"-meaning, your hearing, thinking and responding to the other person's message as well as his response.

- Be very attentive.
- Wait and don't anticipate to answer.
- Let the person or sender finish speaking.
- Don't interrupt. Be a good listener.
- Be calm and don't be emotional even if you hear unpleasant things.
- Provide feedback and ask clarifying questions once in a while. "Do I get your idea?"

Follow a counsel from Apostle James 1:19 NASB when he said "Let everyone be quick to hear, slow to speak and slow to anger." Remember, a sincere prayer is the most direct communication to our loving God.

Emotional Health

> *"Human beings could alter their lives*
> *by altering their attitudes of mind."*
> William James

Every psychological-minded person wants to know the meaning of **emotional health** and its importance to life.

Countless people today are suffering from a severe kind of emotional crisis as shown by the unabated trend of negative aggression i.e. constant domestic bickering, political mudslinging, killings, terrorizing and other destructive upheavals, including all the "psychosomatic" (mind-body) illnesses causes by unresolved emotional conflicts.

Let us then understand our fundamental self-concept. Why are many Filipinos becoming to be oversensitive? Well, this particular reaction basically boils down to their "shaky" or "onion skin" (unstable) kind of emotionality.

What then is emotional health? Psychosocial authorities define emotional health as person's <u>ability to cope with his innate emotions</u>. (It's also synonymous with mental health or wellness.) In life, we sometimes experience for instance, anger, fear, failures, etc. How we handle these feelings determine our emotional nature. But most emotionally stable people can cope well with emotional conflicts. They could work their way through problems in a constructive way.

A person with poor emotional health has trouble handling his emotional disturbance in life. When the problem is too much to bear, the person may lose control. He may try to bury the problem (escape mechanism) by resorting to taking drugs, drinking liquor, destroying things and blaming the whole world for his failures. If things become too unbearable he may resort to committing crimes or may crack-up (breakdown), or may end his life (suicide).

A person who possessed a very sound emotional health evidently manifests by linking who he is and truly accepting himself. We call this as <u>Good Self-Image or Self-Concept</u>. This involves expressing his emotions in a healthy way, facing life's problems and dealing with its pressures.

However, nobody is spared from emotional turmoil, one way or another. We sometimes experience some unpleasant feelings such as anxiety, anger, depression, and fear. However, under ordinary circumstances, these feelings just go away after a while. And more so, if one knows "how to roll with the punches," so to speak. Your ardent prayers will greatly help indeed.

Here are some basic characteristic attitudes that could help greatly in coping with emotional upheavals in life.

- Understand reality and deal with it constructively.
- Adapt a realistic demand for change.
- Be able to cope with stresses.
- Love everyone (including your enemies).
- Be able to work productively.
- Develop your true spirituality (Christ-oriented) life.

Remember that **emotional health** is the quality that enables us to enjoy the good times as well as get through miserable times. A truly emotionally healthy person is said to have come to terms with himself as well as the world around him as we consistently emphasize in our Holistic Therapy sessions.

Basic Psychological Needs

*"Satisfaction in life needs depends not
on the number of years, but on your will."*
Michel de Montaigne

Many of our people are so unaware of the emotional or the psychological needs that are responsible for their efficiency or inefficiency. Psychologists claim that those psychological needs are even more important than material needs. Why? It is because failure to satisfy these needs can disturb man's health and would adversely affect his whole efficiency in life.

Authorities identified <u>six emotional needs of man</u>. Let us learn them:

1. **Man needs love.** Essentially, he needs to love others and be loved. He depends on his fellowmen to survive. He needs others to protect him, to develop him and to make him become a reputable somebody.

2. **The need for security.** Man is secured if he has enough income or resources to buy the necessities of life now and in the future. Another element in security is confidence in one's own ability to solve problems and survive in the face of adversity.

3. **The need for creative expression.** Every man has the need to use his energies and power in creative work. Man can involve himself in the area of agriculture, craftsmanship, or office activity, etc. and woman can engage in the development and enrichment of the home. Both can find true happiness if they fulfill their potential creativity.

4. **The need for recognition.** Psychosocial authorities confirm that sincere praise and recognition are essential to well-being, progress and efficiency of every human being in society. How many sensitive people felt so depressed and finally committed suicide because they

were terribly rejected and suffered strong feeling of bitterness and emptiness which they could not bear anymore? (Despondency)

5. **The need for identity.** Identity means the ability to accept discipline and submission to authority. Both are essential to mental health. Identity also means the ability to accept other people despite their various attitudes. We are all happy if an ordinary citizen would shout: "I AM A FILIPINO. KAYA KO ITO!" (I can do this.)

6. **The need for God.** Man can never bear to live without the divine succor and faith in God-his Creator. Only religion has the power to make the inevitable constraints of morality bearable. True faith in the living God can give real meaning and purpose in life. The strongest spiritual remedy against all the existing evils of this world is to always connect ourselves to God. "God is our refuge and strength, a tested help in times of troubles." (Psalm 46:1 NLT)

Rudyard Kipling, the English poet, when asked what he wants in his dying moment, whispered, "I WANT GOD."

Emergency Survival

Every responsible person in this planet earth should always be aware and should prepare for any inevitable eventuality in this life, and life-threatening situations like typhoon, earthquake, tsunami, fire, disease, etc. which could possibly occur and confront people.

How many of our people have been deplorably victimized, terribly suffered and died untimely because admittedly, they were not trained and were ignorant of what to do during such a severe situation. Those who fortunately survived the overwhelming and unexpected situations were individuals who had some experiences and some training in actual emergency procedures such as risk-reduction, first-aid, and other safety life-saving measures.

In our childhood and adolescent years our parents encouraged us to join the Scouting Movement and learned the basic emergency first aid procedures. We also learned the basic swimming lessons during summer breaks by adept instructors. At least these early trainings could help and guide us what to do in times of disasters that may happen anytime in our life.

Some Useful Tips on what to do during a disaster:

- Always pray and ask God for guidance.
- Be calm. Don't panic. Be alert and watchful.
- Apply your knowledge of the Basic Emergency Aid Procedures.
- Be guided by the news on radio and TV.
- Always be ready with a carry-all container of finger foods, water, flashlights and other necessary things, if "to evacuate" is advised.
- Don't forget to pray for intercession form the Blessed Mary and St. Michael-the angel.

Death Instinct

"We begin to die as soon as we are born,
and the end is linked to the beginning"
Manilius

People are somehow shocked to know when a

prestigious man in the community meets an untimely and violent death. Well, let us ruminate for a while on the mysterious subject of death. The inescapable reality is–– "Nobody will get out of this world alive." Death is an inevitable process to every living creature. However, every mortal being on this planet always desires to live longer and happier. Fulfillment of such an obsession will basically depend on one's lifestyle.

Death instinct theory was conceptualized by the psychoanalyst Sigmund Freud. He claimed that there was a tendency of man to destroy (to kill) and self-destruct himself (suicide). He was impressed by the wanton destructiveness of World War I by the cruelty of many aspects of human behavior. He believed that like animals, man was also driven by an instinct for destruction. He called it as "Thanatopsis." Death instinct operates in opposition to the equally basic life instinct he called "Eros," which has the constructive goal of self-preservation, social unity, and perpetuation of the species. Hence, Freud pictures human life as a theater of opposition in which those two ultimate forces battle for supremacy. Of course, the life drive is more or a dominant force and always win in this tug of war.

Dr. Karl Menninger, an American psychoanalyst, elaborated on the death instinct of man as shown by the actual cases of active and successful suicide. He also proved that death instinct operates in "slow deadly cases" (indirect suicide) as in the case of smoking, drug addition, alcoholism, the martyrs and invite torture (masochism), the criminal who unconsciously seek punishment, the neurotic who enjoys his invalidism, the psychotic who surrenders reality itself; adventurous people who indirectly engage themselves in extremely hazardous or too risky sport activities such as car racing, sky diving, scuba diving, boxing and wrestling, and other death-defying activities where one false move or miscalculation means death.

Statistics of professionals who are high risk of being killed (murdered) are: judges, lawyers, radio announcers, businessmen, politicians and actors.

We have so little time left to prepare ourselves before that "Hour of Departure" scheduled by God...So, let us make everyday the best day as if it were our last.

The Power of Tears

"Jesus wept."
John 11:35 NIV

The above sorrowful scenario happened when Lazarus, the best friend of Jesus, died. This emphasizes the importance of tears in our lives. Definitely, some relief is achieved when one weeps during a grieving situation and carried off by tears which is the "silent language of grief' according to Voltaire.

We, Filipinos, are known to be a sentimental people. We easily cry when we see sad movies, hear nostalgic music or touched by pathetic stories. There are people in our midst who are deeply emotional and could easily burst into tears when they actually experience an unusual or awesome situations like walking through a valley of beautiful flowers or upon seeing a very imposing and majestic mountain peak or a blue serene lake with birds flying over, or perhaps hearing a perfect rendition of "Moonlight Serenade" by Mozart.

What really are tears? According to a reference in the Internet, tears are the liquid product of a process of lachrimation to clean and lubricate the eyes. In a literary sense, it also refers to "crying." Strong emotions, such as sorrow or elation, may lead to crying. Humans are the only mammals who are generally accepted to cry emotional tears. It is interesting to note that some substance und in lachrymal fluids, lycosyme, fight against bacterial infection as part of the immune system.

Here's a beneficial health finding. People who are afraid to let themselves pour forth their painful emotions to tears can trigger such ailments as asthma, migraine and many other psychosomatic illnesses. Reports claimed that some individuals have died because they repressed their emotions. So, don't pent up your emotions and don't fight back your tears, especially in normal grief reactions or intense emotional upheavals. Some patients are relieved with their chronic colds, sinusitis and other respiratory discomforts because they learn to vent their feelings by crying.

I learned by heart a fitting quotation about tears since I was in high school. "Tears are not to be taken as a sign of weakness but of power." They speak more eloquently than ten thousand tongues. They are the messengers of overwhelming grief, of deep contrition and of unspeakable love."

A theologian once said that God is more pleased with a true repentant sinner who weeps than one who just ask forgiveness without any heartfelt feeling at all.

So friends, when sorrow or joy overwhelm you, pour out your precious tears to fully express your deepest sentiments for the sake of your physical, mental, emotional and spiritual well-being.

Steps to Follow in Drinking to Stay Healthy

Most of our body is made up of water. We need it every day to keep our body alive and functioning well. Clean water still remains the best drink we can have. Other drinks that are good for us are fresh fruits and vegetable juices and milk. Some people love to take coffee or tea. These are stimulating beverages. However, they both contain substances that can be harmful when taken in excess. For instance, they can disturb the heart, raise the blood pressure and upset the normal blood flow or pregnant women and adversely affect women's fertility.

To drink healthily:

- Drink clean water. (An average of 8 glasses a day for adults.) Elderlies are advised to take more-10 to 12 glasses a day to benefit their kidneys.
- Limit your intake of coffee or tea to 2 cups (AM & PM) a day.
- If you drink alcohol, drink in moderation (no more than one or two drinks a day...social drinking).
- Take fruit or vegetable juices rather than soft drinks, which are artificially colored and sweetened and carbonated.
- Discover the wide range of delicious herbal teas.
- Take a glass of milk a day for stronger bones. Always drink for your health if you want to live long.

The Benefits of Hard Work

*"Work is the grand curve of
all the maladies and Miseries
that ever beset mankind."*
Thomas Carlyle

If our hero, Dr. Jose Rizal, were alive today, I'm sure, he should have rewritten his fiery novels and should have never used the derogatory word as "indolence" anymore, most especially if he would have known that our domestic helpers and caregivers were consistently earning a great name for themselves as "most industrious and efficient (exportable) workers in the whole world."

Today, there are still a lot of people who view work negatively and see it as something that wears you down, that it produces mental and physical fatigue, and that it produces stress, ill health and early death. It does not mean that man should avoid work because work is stressful. No sir, certainly not. No less than Dr. Hans Selye, the guro on stress, has positively identified in his research that work isn't bad for anybody. He said, "There is more to life than just work. One should work to live, not live to work." According to him, "Positive activities like a pleasant work, wholesome exercise, profitable hobby, good sex, are the 'Spice of Life.'" But the worse that can happen to mankind is only by people never doing anything and just wasting their time in some unimportant activities as experienced by the truly lazy ones.

Work is what authorities say what we have to do. Play is what we like to do. Such simple tasks as gardening, fishing, washing vehicles, and even playing basketball, singing, dancing, etc. is work when you do it for a living. A certain philosopher once said: "Man's characteristic feature is not his wisdom but his constant urge to improve his environment and himself." Hence, man has got to work to improve, meaning to find the kind of work that suits him best, a worthwhile activity that he likes and respect, which is within his talent or capacity.

Examples of great men who were known as hard workers who lived to an advanced age of 89 and 90 were Emilio Aguinaldo, Winston Churchill, Albert Schweitzer, Conrad Adenawer, Charles de Gaul and Pablo Picasso. All of them lived a life of intense activity with "Leisure" by working consistently at what they like to do. They were all self-fulfilled in their own fields of endeavor.

Let us try to emulate them no matter how hard the work is for this is what God wants us all to do while we are still alive and have the energy to perform useful work. Say a prayer to St. Joseph, the laborer and patron saint of good workers.

Warning on Herbal Medicines

"Even (the innocuous) water when taken too much will become harmful (water toxicity)."

Anonymous

Apparently, there is truth to the above saying when applied to taking things indiscriminately without any control at all or without proper regulations. When medical doctors prescribe medicines, they see to it that the dose must be properly determined or regulated to be fully effective and can really cure the disease. Hence, medical authorities, warn people in the indiscriminate use of herbal medicines in place of the ethically approved and prescribed pharmaceutical medicines.

Today, there are a growing number of Filipinos who are taking blindly herbal medicines. Probably because of the rampant advertisement over the mass media (radio, TV. Magazines, etc.). However, people should realize that these herbal products are still unregulated and no one is assured of its safety and equally especially when its package has a very limited content information. Not because it is natural or herbal means it is already safe. No Sir. Herbal supplements are just supplements and they do not provide the proven therapeutic properties. Get this straight please.

Medical reports warn that the long range intake of herbal medicine may bring serious damage especially to the liver and kidney functions as bared by the National Kidney Institute of the Philippines. In 2004, there were 5,900 Filipinos who underwent dialysis. These figures, as reports further claimed, has continually increased in the past four or more years by 10%. Herbal medicines may bring damage to one's kidney. This could lead to dialysis which is very expensive at P25,000 or more a month or a kidney transplant which average costs half a million pesos. Hence, herbal medicines must be studied carefully first before purchasing and taking them indiscriminately. Some kidney symptoms induced by herbal medicines include hypertension, kidney stones, urinary retention, urinary tract carcinoma, among others, as reported factually.

Nowadays, a lot of people are using mostly the common dietary herbs which have been used safely for quite some time, such as spices i.e. onions, ginger, garlic, and the well-known, green tea, tomatoes, grape-seed extract, honey, oils and other essential extracts from fruits and vegetables. These are all approved supplements. However, authorities are questioning the newer, exoteric-termed herbal preparations, using strange and funny sounding names. Herbal manufacturers are apparently using paid charlatans who blurt all over the radio, convincing innocent and gullible people of their so-called "cure all" products from tumors to cancers. Can you believe these blatant claims? Preposterous! Some say this is "Faith Healing" (due to purely psychological effect) or "Fake Healing."

Well, you be the judge. In this country, when you die, whether you take herbs or not, nobody will ever question. It's always your own choice, man! (Democracy?)

The Rare Gift of Psychic Power

Fr. Jaime Bulatao, a well-known Atenean Psychologists who used to give the residents in Psychiatry at the UP-PGH Medical Center in Manila years ago on the interesting topic of Psychic Phenomena. All were amazed with the valuable discoveries of psychic powers that could benefit mankind, if fully developed and properly harnessed.

When we talk about "psychic," we mean a person who possesses supernatural powers. **Parapsychology** is the study of psychic phenomena. **Extra Sensory Perception** (ESP) is the reception of information by non-sensory means, not involving the 5 senses light sight, hearing, smell, taste and touch. **Psychokinesis (PK)** is the exercise of direct mental influence over a physical object or process. Example: A person with "PK" is able to "will" the dice to come to rest at a desired number. **Deja vu,** is the feeling that one has seen or experienced something happening in the present or at some previous time. There are persons who experience unusual state of which they claim that they were able to see the place before even if they have not actually seen the place.

Another psychic gift of some is the ability to predict events in the future. For instance, the crash of an American Airline where hundreds died at the O'Hare Airport in Chicago, USA, was accurately predicted by a psychic. This is known as **precognition.**

Scientific researches in USA have evidently proven the true happening of psychic phenomena in the world. It is claimed that the Russian researchers are more advanced in terms of psychic phenomena. Uri Geller incredibly demonstrated his psychic feat when he bended metal spoons with his powerful gaze, a psychokinesis power!

Our Filipino Psychic Surgeon Agpawa from Baguio City successfully operated our local and foreign clients through his powerful psychic hands.

Teresita Basa from Dumaguete City who was murdered in Chicago, USA, was able to reveal her real murderer through a co-worker whom she used as a medium, by identifying the true murderer.

Reports of amazing psychic power are coming up. Hopefully, science will be able to harness the valuable process or tool of psychic power to help mankind solve his various problems.

Understanding Your Feelings

All living creatures are believed to have feelings, a tangible sign of life. Plants "bleed" when they are wounded. Some move with the sun as the sunflowers. Some show sensitiveness when touched, like some mimosas or touch-me-nots. Porpoises "cry" when they are killed. Most wild animals "cuddle" their young. Man, the highest rational being, ironically speaking, is the only creature who kills the innocent fetus through abortion. I am shocked to know this fact from authorities. And yet the wildest animals in the jungle never kill their off springs. They still have their maternal feelings called "instinctual care". We cannot always blame Satan for this behavior for we have free will to reckon with. So, don't blame the authors of this Reproductive Health Bill. We always use our conscience and freedom of choice. If we are true Christians, then we should never kill.

In psychiatry, we are so much concerned particularly in our patient's serious feelings of despair (depression) which unknowingly may lead to a very unfortunate event–– suicide. So, it is very important to know the different degrees of depression in order to prevent self-destruction.

Normal depression. This is the most common feeling of sadness, disappointment, despair, frustration of unhappiness. These are the universal experiences of most people in daily life which are a normal feeling state.

Grief or uncomplicated bereavements. Grief reaction is a normal, appropriate, affective sadness in response to a recognizable loss. For instance, a death in the family or loss of some valuable things like a burned house, health or wealth as in bankruptcy, etc. of which one will grieve or lament. However, these feelings are only temporary and one can recover in time. This reaction is self-limiting and gradually subsides.

Mild depression. We call this in psychiatry as "dysthymic disorder". This occurs when the cause is less obvious than in normal grief or the depression is more severe. The individual usually realizes that the response is excessive but does not recognize the underlying cause.

Major depression. This is a more severe form of

depression characterized by a depressed, anxious and irritable mood, loss or gain in weight, loss of interest in normal activities, poor sleep pattern, feelings agitated or slowed down, depressed sex drive, physical aches or pains, feelings of worthlessness, feeling of guilt, poor concentration or lack of ability to think, recurrent thought of death or suicide.

Psychologists generally classify emotion into four primary feelings namely: *sadness, happiness, fears, and anger with auxiliary feelings of each.* We have just to call our feelings as "pleasant" or "unpleasant" and to understand and resolve them so we can peacefully and constructively live.

Abreaction-A Good Tool for Pent-up Emotion

A very important instrument that psychiatrists often use in helping dissipate a bottled-up or long repressed negative emotion is "catharsis." Clinical Psychologists also call this as "abreaction."

Psychiatrists, psychologists, as well as sociologists have consistently reported that most people in a highly urbanized and civilized society have been suffering from deep and hidden unresolved anger, hostility, resentment and other forms of indifferences or antagonisms towards their kin, relatives and neighbors. The unresolved negative feelings are the major causes of serious conflicts and stresses in life. All these antagonistic feelings, if kept and repressed for a long time, would be the main etiological roots of many psychosomatic illnesses in this world. Countless of people from all walks of life have filled up the hospitals with their complaints of stomach ulcers, bronchial asthma, hypertension, chest and joint pains, palpitations, sleeplessness, obesity, lack of appetite and other complaints where the doctors found no positive cause of their perennial and recurrent complaints.

The psychiatric treatment for all the repressed negative physical and emotional conflicts is known as **psychotherapy.** Catharsis is one of the major instruments treating neurotic patients. Psychologists generally call this instrument as **abreaction.**

Catharsis or abreaction is a psychoanalytic therapy wherein the client or patient is made to verbalize, express or react with adequate emotionality and revive the repressed forgotten memories or experiences with full expression of the associated pent-up effects. Trained counselors usually use this therapy in their counseling to let the clients fully express their bottled-up emotions.

Psychiatrists say that **repression** is bad for it affects the nervous system. The deadly psychosomatic illnesses like heart attack, stroke, bleeding ulcers and other chronic and deadly diseases would result.

In the Sacrament of Reconciliation, the emotional feelings of the penitent, after a sincere confession to his confessor, become so therapeutic, there is so much peace in his soul and whole being!

What One Must Do During a Heart Attack

Heart attack occurs when a blood supply in a part of heart muscles is blocked by a blood clot in a coronary artery.

I got a very useful information-a brief summary by a cardiologist on how to help a person who is having a "heart attack."

If you are a responsible adult who happen to be in an

emergency, don't panic but pray and render a "heroic act" by doing the following procedures:

1. Clear people who overcrowd the patient; he needs all the oxygen to breathe.
2. Let someone immediately call for an ambulance.
3. Do not move patient.
4. Keep patient in semi-sitting position.
5. Open collar, loosen tie and belt.
6. Encourage deep breathing.
7. Give patient medication which he may have in his position (if he has had previous attacks) but do not use this medication if the patient is in state of shock or unconsciousness after acute coronary closure. The result may be disastrous. Hence, use nitroglycerin and other related medications with extreme reservation or seek immediate professional advice, if possible.

If heart stops beating, use "closed method" cardiac massage (Cardio Resuscitation):

1. Place patient flat on his back.
2. Kneel and straddle patient.
3. Place heel of palm of right hand on patient's breastbone.
4. Place left hand over your right hand and push down so that the breastbone is depressed about one (1) inch.
5. Release.
6. Repeat this every 1-2 seconds for at least 10 minutes or until heartbeat and breathing are resumed.
7. If someone else is also available, have him

render mouth-to-mouth artificial respiration at the same time that you are conducting cardiac massage.

WARNING!

Patient with coronary heart disease requires hospital care. Seek the help of cardiologist. Unfortunately, a lot of Filipinos who are called to assist a victim who is in the state of shock or unconsciousness immediately would resort to their old crude procedure locally called as "dapin-on" (putting a pressure on the pit of the stomach to stop the "kabuhi" from pulsating. This is a wrong procedure to apply.

Prevention and Control of Contagious Diseases

Inevitably, outbreak of communicable diseases will always happen in any part of the world despite the advent of modem preventive measures. For instance, AIDS--Acquired Immune Deficiency Syndrome has been known to us only these few decades ago. Another deadly viral infection is **EBOLA,** which has been killing a lot of people in Africa and in the neighboring countries. Another recent respiratory contagious disease is **MERS** COV-Middle East Respiratory Syndrome Coronavirus, which is widely spreading in South Korea so much so that health authorities are having a hard time controlling it.

A few people know about the worst and uncontrolled pandemic of influenza that spread throughout the world in the 18th century where millions of people died.

It is really imperative that people of all ages must know and learn how to prevent the spread of a communicable disease. Such simple ways which can be practiced at home are as follows:

1. Avoid spitting anywhere. This is one of the effective ways of spreading harmful microbes or germs.
2. Always observe proper hygiene; strictly teach everyone in the household proper health procedures such as hand washing, etc.
3. Don't forget to cover your nose when you sneeze and mouth when you cough. Always bring a handkerchief or tissue for your use. Dispose your sputum in a proper receptacle.
4. Avoid overcrowding.
5. Keep room well ventilated and clean.
6. Illnesses should be considered contagious until proper diagnosis is definitely established.
7. At the first sign of illness the patient should be isolated and to separate his linens and utensils.
8. The sick should be attended to and treated at once.
9. Patient should be referred to a Medical Internist if symptoms may not respond well to your initial medications.
10. Patient may need laboratory work-up to establish the true diagnosis as well as treatment.

Remember: Cleanliness is next to Godliness!

Humor-A Healthy Emotional Outlet

One of the cheapest and most available sources of happiness in this world is laughter. The sense of humor is a God-given gift. He wants us to taste a glimpse of heaven which the Holy Bible describes as a "place of perpetual cheerfulness." According to the Reader's Digest-"Laughter is the best medicine." Humor is truly considered to be one of the antidotes for stressful living, a good tonic for boredom and a safety value for mental breakdown.

Humor is aptly defined by the dictionary as a person's temperament, mood, and state of mind, whim, fancy, caprice, comicality, and the ability to appreciate or express what is funny, amusing or ludicrous.

What then is the psychological function of humor in our life? Let us take for instance, the following situations. Laughing for example, at the weak points or people in authority, enables us to express hostility safely and without fear of retaliation. This subtle mechanism by indirectly hitting or criticizing the so-called "reputable individuals" in our society like politicians or some others who have committed big blunders in their lives, say corruption, is being utilized by some radio commentators in expressing their shameful acts in the air by exposing them in a joking manner without naming names and done in a subtle way or with an excuse like-"sabi ng duwende, daw!" (According to a leprechaun.) It's very effective indeed.

Psychologists say that laughing with others increases our sense of solidarity, unity and acceptance. Getting the point of a joke enhances self-confidence. By taking serious things jokingly fortifies our sense of perspectives. The act of laughing itself provides a healthy release of pent-up or repressed emotional energy, especially when one is beset with a lot of tensions and stresses in one's life. It is really true that a person who belly laughs rarely belly aches.

A natural humorist or a comedian is a person who has a well-developed sense of humor. A good joke is something everyone appreciates and enjoys in other people. An occasional hearty laugh actually lightens the burdens of life considerably and enables us to overcome some difficulties in our lives. Studies have shown that those who have a good sense of humor are less inclined to suffer from ulcers and high blood pressure. Humor brings people closer together and helps people relax. Many of us like to listen to speakers such as politicians, teachers, priests and others who know how to inject humorous stories, jokes and funny anecdotes to their topics. It is never boring to hear them talk. To tell a joke that would really make people laugh is an art in itself.

My late father, Andoy, was fund of joking and many of his jokes were taken from his actual life experiences as a biology teacher and that's why they were so effective. In my class in psychiatry before, which was 1 o'clock in the afternoon, most of my students managed to attend the very unholy hour because of my selected jokes, which helped them keep awake.

World famous comedians like Bob Hope, Red Skelton, and our famous Dolphy are all emotionally mature people because they can laugh about their personal weaknesses. Unfortunately, there are some individuals who are humorless and too serious in their outlook in life that they are like salads without any dressing at all. Remember the saying that "the world laughs with you when you are happy but when you cry, you cry alone." God wants us to be happy my friends, in the right way of course.

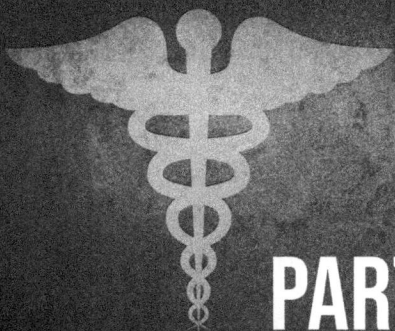

PART VII

STRESS AND OTHER MENTAL DISORDERS

Stress Kills!

> *"Prayer, faith and love are the most powerful weapon against stress."*
> Dr. Bernie S. Siegel

Today, modern man is inevitably beset by both internal and external stresses. His life is full of hastes, worry, frustrations, anxiety, fear, tension, pain and pressures. All these Are caused by uncontrollable phase and demands of contemporary times arising from rapid social, technological and unpredictable environmental changes and crisis situations perceived as threatening, and therefore, causing undue insecurities affected by stress. It is an inescapable reality and phenomena of life.

Reports claim that millions of people from all walks of life are suffering from 'stress-related disorders" such as high blood pressure, sudden heart attacks, stroke, bleeding, stomach ulcers, kidney troubles, cancers, family discords, suicide, nervous breakdowns, and a host of psychosomatic illnesses which are brought about by various stresses of this 2P[1] century. Stress is the No. 1 health enemy. Hence, it's very important to know and learn how to cope up with everyday stress to be able to survive its devastating effects of disease and death.

What then is stress? Authorities define stress as "a chronically high level of mental arousal and bodily tension that exceeds a person's capacity to cope, resulting in distress, disease and death."

Mental hygienists said that stress becomes dangerous when it is intense, unduly prolonged, uncontrolled and affects a particular organ of the body. Dr. Hans Selye, a guru on stress strongly suggests that one should strive to reach a state of "oustress" or optimum stress level, which is healthy and agreeable response to stress.

There are three major responses or reactions of our body to stress, namely:

A. Physical responses. For example: cold sweats, diarrhea, rapid heart-beat, easily fatigued, shortness of breath, headaches, weakness, dizziness, restlessness, emotional instability.

B. Psychological responses. Example: poor concentration, difficulty in making decisions, loss of self-confidence, irritability, worry or anxiety, depression, irrational fear or panic behavior.

C. Behavioral responses. Example: smoking, drinking or taking drugs, increased used of medications, nail-biting, and other mannerisms, accident proneness, insomnia, nightmares, loss or increase of appetite, reckless driving, uncalled for aggressiveness.

Psychiatrists said that unexpressed emotions

whether positive or negative, frequently cause stress and becomes conditioned or fixed. If a stressor persists and no intervention is done, then the "exhaustion stage" occurs, the damage to the organ-system is irreparable and death results.

Strategies for stress management:

1. Build up your general health (proper diet, rest, exercise, relaxation techniques and other positive health practices).
2. Change the situation (source of stress).
3. Change your attitude (perception on stress).
4. Change your bodily state (learn to substitute relaxation responses for stress responses).

Most of all, cultivate an authentic Christian qualities- prayerfulness, forgiveness, love, mildness and patience. Put God first in your life, my friend.

Bust Stress, Stay Healthy and Live Longer

"In my distress, I cried out to the Lord and He heard me, my cry reach His ears."
Holy Scripture

Anti-stress authorities said that holidays like Christmas, despite its merrymakings, are also considered stressful moments. Below are some effective ways in alleviating negative stress reactions in our hectic life. These selected ways could help you function better and live longer, that is, if you follow them well:

1. CHANGE YOUR ATTITUDE. Learn to look at things positively. Stop useless worrying, forgive

offenses, be moderate in all activities, learn to say NO and be happy.

2. WATCH YOUR DIET. A well-balanced diet (good nutrition), a variety of vegetables, fresh fruits, low carbohydrates and fat, high protein and fiber diet, eat more fish than animal meat, low salt and sugar. Eat less. Take vitamin supplements and minerals when needed.

3. EXERCISE MODERATELY. This is a must to keep fit, strong and healthy. Aerobics, like brisk walking, is proven to be good for your heart and other body organs.

4. GET ADEQUATE SLEEP, REST AND RELAXATION. Be sure to sleep an average of 6 to 8 hours at night. A 30-minute catnap is found to be beneficial to most people. An elderly needs an hour rest in the afternoon.

5. MANAGE YOUR TIME WELL. Prevent time wasters-long TV shows, chatting needlessly, etc. Avoid procrastination, too. Do your priorities first.

6. BE CALM AND SLOW DOWN. Never rush doing things. Walk calmly, eat slowly, and don't talk so rapidly. Shun workaholism. Don't suffer "Bum-Out Syndrome" and die early.

7. EXPRESS AND CONTROL YOUR ANGER. This is a healthy outlet for your pent-up emotion. Psychologists suggest the use of punching bag for the quiet men to vent hidden hostile feelings. Women can well verbalize their feelings.

8. AVOID HARMFUL HABITS AND POLLUTIONS. Such vices like smoking, heavy drinking, abusing drugs, womanizing, excessive eating,

gambling, are injurious activities and will lead to early death. Avoid pollutants from air, food, water and environment.

9. LAUGH AT YOURSELF. Laughter is proven to be the best medicine.

10. STAY OUT OF BAD DEBTS. Money is not bad but love of money is evil. A lot of people in our society today are too obsessed with wealth. They want to get rich quick and keep up with the Joneses. But once they become broke, they panic and suffer extreme insecurity and land in the hospital. So budget well and live within your means.

11. LISTEN TO MELODIOUS MUSIC. Music is a great relaxant for it stimulates good response of your muscles, brain and nerves. Try to listening to soothing and relaxing music.

12. TAKE A VACATION. This will provide a break in the vicious pattern of your hectic or competitive routine of your work. Make your vacation restful and enjoyable.

13. HAVE A REGULAR MEDICAL CHECK-UP AND SEEK PROFESSIONAL HELP. This will determine whether your physical or mental set is alright or not. Remember, "An ounce of prevention is worth a pound of cure." Psychotherapy can help resolve deep-seated conflicts that may cause a lot of stress, which shortens your life span.

14. FOR DAILY LIVING. Maintain a strong faith, be prayerful, read the Holy Scriptures, receive the sacraments, serve your church and community well. Never neglect your poorest neighbors. Be an authentic Christian. Let GOD control your life, my friend.

The Best Kind of Attitude in dealing with Stress in Life

I have just found a beautiful and popular message that has been circulated via email so often. It is a very inspirational message for it pursues realistic goals that are meaningful and inspiring to everyone. It appropriately describes the kind of attitude we can develop in dealing with Stress in our life. I would like to share and highly recommend that you make a copy of this beautiful message and read it regularly to give you and your love ones a daily dose of lasting inspiration and hopefully will help you distress your life.

When the door of happiness closes, another opens; but often times will look so long at the closed door that we don't see the one which has been opened for us.

Dream what you want to dream; go where you want to go; be what you want to be, because you have only one life and one chance to do all the things you want to do.

May you have enough happiness to make you sweet, enough trials to make you strong, enough sorrow to keep you human and enough hope to make you happy.

The happiest of people don't necessarily have the best of everything; they just make the most of everything that comes their way.

The brightest future will always be based on a forgotten past; you can't go forward in life until you let go of your past failures and heartaches.

When you were born, you were crying and everyone around you was smiling. Live your life so at the end, you're the one who is smiling and everyone around you is crying.

Don't count the years--count the memories...Life

is not measured by the breaths we take but by the moments that we take our breath away!

Stress is something we have to live with, but also something we can utilize to live fully.

PTSD-Post-Traumatic Stress Disorder

"Crisis when they occur have at least this advantage that they force us to think."
Jawaharlal Nehru

In the last past weeks, typhoons Ondoy and Pepeng brought a terrible havoc to our people in Luzon. Everyone–– rich or poor, young and old were not spared and they all suffered an extremely severe traumatic experience in their lives. Many people lost their lives, properties and other precious possessions just in a few days.

The above terrifying scenario has subjected unprepared people to what is known as Post Traumatic stress Disorder (PTSD). This most unpleasant stress disorder is caused by experiencing a severe psychic trauma. **Psychic trauma** is defined as an inescapable event that overwhelms an individual's existing coping mechanism. The stressors in PTSD could be markedly distressing to anyone and experience intense fear, terror and helplessness. Such gruesome situations experienced as being brutally raped or assaulted; in bloody hand-to-hand combat; severely tortured in death camps; continuous bombing; trapped for several days in a deep mining tunnel; and other severe life-threatening situations in life.

Symptoms of PTSD. There are three:

1. Those suffering from it repeatedly relive (re-experience) the traumatic experience. This may be through flashbacks, intrusive thoughts, memories, nightmares, or intense emotional and physical reactions to reminders of the event.
2. Avoidance and emotional numbing. That is, the person loses interest and withdraws from people and ordinary life.
3. An increased emotional arousal. The sufferers may be easily startled or have difficulty getting sleep, irritable, or angry outburst. PTSD may also trigger physical complaints such as headaches, digestive problems, chest pains, dizziness or vertigo, may go more visit to the doctor. These may be psychosomatic disorders.

Who is at the greatest risk? Not everyone exposed to extremely trauma gets PTSD. Factors such as (1) the severity of the trauma, (2) proximity to the event, (3) the duration of the experience, (4) the degree of danger involved. This is the reason why people involved in the military warfare, terrifying combat and prisoner of war and victims of international violence are at the greatest risks of developing PTSD. A past history of extreme trauma such as rape or childhood abuse also increase vulnerability to PTSD. This includes people who survived or witnessed the harrowing attack, lost their loved ones or were involved in the rescue and recovery efforts.

Effective treatment depends on how early the intervention would be. The sooner the treatment is sought the better the chance of recovery. When PTSD is untreated, it can become more disabling and it may be accompanied by chronic anxiety, severe phobia and depression.

Management:

- <u>Psychotherapy</u> by a professional therapist is needed a lot. Cognitive-behavior therapy-helping the patient adopt healthier ways of coping with emotional crisis.
- <u>Relaxation technique</u>. To be guided by an experienced therapist or a self-help relaxation process.
- <u>Medication</u>. Judicious use of some anti-anxiety and antidepressant agents.
- <u>Spiritual therapy</u>. Prayers can definitely reduce stress and has a calming effect. Let your prayers be a life preserver.

Here's a powerful scriptural verse in time of calamity-"Let us not fear, though the Earth gives way, the mountain fall, the waters roar and foam for God is our refuge and strength ever present in time of trouble." (Psalm 40:1-3)

Depression

"Untreated depression can be
as much a killer as cancer."
Fr. Andrew Page

For decades, a vast majority of our people always have the belief that depression is just a part of passing sadness in life. However, the research finding of depression points to the fact that it involves changes in brain chemicals (neurotransmitters). Hence, an uncontrolled and untreated depression could seriously devastate even the brightest individuals who suddenly commit suicide.

In fact, I know of bright seminarians, three clergies, a Bishop from Pakistan and even psychiatrists abroad who were severely depressed and even committed suicide. This shows that no matter how religious and bright a person is, he is still vulnerable to severe depression, which leads to suicide.

It pays to know depression as a serious illness so that we can identify, prevent its occurrence, and know what to do when it hits us.

Depression is a common psychological condition characterized by sadness, gloom, dejection, and despondency, which may lead to suicide if not timely intervened.

SIGNS OF DEPRESSION:

People suffering from depression usually feel unhappy and lose interest in their work, and hobbies or in normal activities they used to enjoy. They also:

- Feel worthless, guilty, helpless, or hopeless (despondency)
- Have trouble sleeping or sleep too much
- Loss appetite or may over-eat (a cover up)
- Feel tired, weakened, and has low energy
- Feel restless, anxious, and irritable
- Poor concentration, forgetful, or unable to make a decision
- Lost interest in sex
- Think or talk about death

(Any three of the above criteria means serious depression.) Plus-other physical symptoms such as headache, stomachache, backache, which may also be signs of depression.

CAUSES:

The primary cause of depression has been found to be due to imbalance of the neurotransmitters (i.e. serotine) in the brain. Depression could be triggered by such factors as:

- Genetic (hereditary)
- Stressful life events (i.e. financial economic upheavals)
- Personal loss of loved object (i.e. death of a loved one, break up of close relationship, or other meaningful losses)
- Trauma in childhood–– abandonment, etc.
- Physical illness-stroke, cancer, AIDS, etc.
- Medications for hypertension, heart medications, and some pain medications
- Drugs or alcohol abuse causes chemical imbalance in the brain
- Hormones-its deficiency such as hypothyroidism and menopause in women causing depression

TREATMENT:

A. Seek early professional help before it's too late (psychiatrists can judiciously prescribe effective antidepressant pills to stabilize the impaired mood. Plus counselling sessions to prevent recurrence.
B. May need hospitalization for severe cases.
C. Other sources of help. Don't bottle-up but verbalize and confide your inner feelings (problems) to a level-headed person like a

close friend, family members and mature neighbor.

D. Talk to your counselor, a priest, minister who may be trained in crisis intervention.

Strong Indicators for High Risks to Commit Suicide

Here are the high risk factors for suicide:

1. Presence of a Suicide Plan in mind.
2. Presence of recurring depression.
3. History of Suicide in the family.
4. History of suicidal attempt.
5. Unresolved personal conflicts, example: Jilted or rejected, unresolved homosexuality, loss of loved one, etc.
6. Drug abuse, alcoholism, presence of chronic disease and constant pain, terminal illness, extreme humiliation.
7. High achievers with perfectionist personality; inability to cope with success; failures, etc.
8. Suffering from mental disorders: Example-- Affective or Bipolar Impulsive behavior, accident prone, etc.
9. Utter lack of faith and emotionally unstable personality, over sensitive, struggling with severe stresses.
10. The person maybe keeping potential deadly objects like rope, sharp blade, a gun, poison, or a "goodbye letter" hidden somewhere in the room.

One must be a very warm and sincere person to

win the trust and confidence of the despondent who is silently crying for help.

The Psychology of Insecurity

Undoubtedly, everyone in this world ultimately desired to attain a state of security in many ways; physically, mentally, emotionally, socially and spiritually. The person who has the best chance of achieving these valuable qualities is one who possesses a stable and mature personality with such desirable traits as-loving, honest, kind, diligent, consistent, considerate and God-fearing person.

Let us then take up a typical example of an extremely insecure person known to man. (We are not talking about economic security here.) It is indeed very ironic that this person who became a subtle victim of insecurity happens to belong to a well-known family in the city. He has attained a higher degree of education, married, a professional with a prestigious position in society and professed to be a Christian. However, he has a very negative attitude in life. Apparently, he possesses a very repulsive character. He is egoistic, indifferent, hostile, vindictive, secretive, suspicious and an extremely manipulative person. He had been observed by his colleagues to have no friends except, perhaps, for a few with odious traits. In fact, this guy wears a bullet-proof vest when he goes out of his house–– a tangible sign of a strong insecurity feeling and a paranoid thought that he might be shot anytime. This is a classic example of a very insecure person.

I will cite concrete manifestations of marked insecurity feelings among our people:

1. The building of high walls around the house and laden with broken glasses or rolls of barb wires.
2. Keeping of ferocious watchdogs like German Shepherds or Dobermans or any barking dogs to guard the house.
3. Hiring of security guards.
4. Placing a hidden door bell near the main gate.
5. Cars are heavily tinted with black color.
6. Wearing of hat, dark goggles or helmets to camouflage identity.
7. Wearing of bullet-proof vest for protection.
8. Husband or wife may secretly hire private detective to detect any foul play of either spouse.
9. Buying of a weapon (shotgun) to be used against possible intruders.
10. A paranoid husband installed electric wires around their house but unfortunately, accidentally electrocuted his teenage son who comes home late at night from a party.

Christmas time is the most precious moment to rejoice for the Holy Redeemer who is born to give PEACE and JOY to mankind. (A message of true security and freedom from harm.) Hence, Christmas is the time when all adversaries lay down their arms (ceasefire) and duly respect the sacred tidings gladly sang by the Angels: "Let there be peace to men of goodwill!"

How ironic indeed that there are still the so-called "Christians" who never respect this very Season of Love and Peace but still go on with their evil and scheming intentions.

Anxiety-The Hidden Emotion

"Nothing in life is to be feared.
It is only to be understood."

Marie Curie

Today, we are not living in an "Age of Anxiety." Anxiety is the most common unavoidable emotional disturbance in our stress-laden society. Every time a person wakes up in the morning, up to the time he goes to bed at night, he experiences a bit of anxiety, one way or another.

We often hear clergies delivering sermons in church saying, "Deliver us from useless anxiety, O Lord." This is to emphasize the fact that people worry so much, but statistics show that 92% of their worries are just imagined problems and never happened at all and the 8% is manageable. Worry, someone said, is like a rocking chair. It keeps on moving but it does not bring you anywhere.

What then is anxiety? The dictionary defines it as: uneasiness, worry, apprehension, tension, distress, dread, or fear. Psychiatrists define anxiety as an emotion that a person experiences in the face of a perceived threat of danger. It is called "perceived" because the threat or danger can be real or imagined. If the danger is real, then anxiety can serve as a positive warning device and therefore it becomes a useful defense that can protect a person from harm. However, if the anxiety is imagined (existing only in the mind) then it becomes a negative baggage, a useless one for it makes a person down, saps his energy and would make him a crippled person and ineffective (an imaginary invalid).

Summarily, some manifestations of anxiety in various severity are: feeling shaky or restlessness, tense, chest discomfort, rapid heartbeat, high blood pressure, shortness of breath, tremors, sweating, urge to urinate, pallor, irritable, sleeplessness, poor appetite, easily rattled, impaired sexual functions, fear of getting crazy and fear of dying, etc. If one suffers from any four (4) of these symptoms, then, he is suffering from anxiety.

If anxiety becomes uncontrollable, it may lead to panic attack-the height of anxiety. Worse, if this becomes extreme and uncontrollable, it will now lead to a serious mental breakdown known as "psychosis" (insanity to laymen). This illness, however, is very much treatable if managed early and adequately.

The general approaches to the treatment of anxiety disorders are:

1. Medical Approach. Judicious use of minor tranquilizers. Caution: These are habit-forming drugs.
2. Psychotherapy. Done by trained and experienced psychotherapists (psychiatrists).
3. Behavioral Approach. By licensed clinical psychologists. Use of relaxation technique, desensitization, flooding, etc.
4. Common Sense Approach. Proper diet, exercise, sleep, recreation, no vices, balance lifestyle.
5. Spiritual Approach. Effective prayers, meditation, reading of Holy Scriptures (Bible), etc. Here is a consoling biblical verse for anxious people: "Even though I walk through the valley of the shadow of death, I fear no evil for you are with me. Your rod and your staff, they comfort me." (Psalm 23)

Know Common Psychiatric Emergencies

One of the most life-threatening emergencies is suicide, a major source of death. Unfortunately, many psychiatric emergencies are not recognized by most people for the potential harm that they may cause.

Just like a bolt of lightning that strikes in a clear blue sky, many of these untreated mentally and emotionally disturbed patients suffer from an uncontrollable frenzy of violent behavior that may inevitably result to death of innocent people or destruction of precious properties. Definitely, this occurrence is a great source of extreme anxiety or panic in the whole community.

Actually to a layman, a psychiatric emergency is simply the sudden appearance of unusual disordered or socially inappropriate behavior. Psychiatrists define Psychiatric Emergency as a disturbance in thoughts (ideas), feelings (emotion) or actions (behavior) for which immediate treatment is deemed necessary.

Let me just mention some common psychiatric emergencies. (The lengthy causes and symptoms are purposely omitted for lack of space herein.)

1. Acute psychotic states such as schizophrenic turmoil, delusional or paranoid ideation.
2. Acute anxiety or panic reaction.
3. Suicidal behavior in extremely depressed persons.
4. Severe agitation and violence, quarrels, actual fight, manifesting extreme rage and aggression.
5. Toxic alcoholic and drug withdrawal reactions.
6. Epileptic furor (i.e. temporal love epilepsy) and cerebral diseases.

7. Post-partum (after delivery) and post-operative reactions.
8. Endocrine crisis (i.e. Hypoglycemia).
9. Manic or hypo manic states in affective (mood) disorders.
10. Infective conditions (i.e. violent delirious states) and others.

In terms of treatment of psychiatric emergencies, it really needs a competent psychiatrist to manage such a highly uncontrollable mental and emotional condition for it entails the judicious use of specific therapeutic agents such as anti-anxiety, antipsychotic and appropriate psychological maneuvers to successfully control and effect a cure.

Therefore, the recognition of psychiatric emergencies is very important before effective management can be achieved and help improve the quality of cure these horrifying mental and emotional disturbances bring.

LIVE! It does not pay to just Worry

"A useless life is an early death."

Goethe

In our transitory sojourn in this world, I would like to share with you a few highly esteemed values that are worth achieving in this life before we finally return to dust.

1. Live the present moment. Living the present moment frees our mind from guilt, anxiety, and regrets. The past is past and we don't know

the future. God knows what to do with every moment of our lives.

2. <u>It does not pay to worry</u>. Worry does not accomplish anything except to lose our appetite, sleep and zest for living. It does not solve any problem and it only destroys our peace of mind. If we just have enough patience, couples with our ardent prayers, things get resolved.

3. <u>We have to endure our forsakenness.</u> Accept that life is now what we want it to be. Life is a mixture of good as well as bad times. It is a test and it is a tough one. But for those who know how to ride and adjust, survive.

4. <u>Be first to love</u>. This is very difficult to do for those who are offended. But Christ explicitly said, "Love your enemy. In reality, if we truly forgive and love our enemy, we will be greatly relieved form the burden of guilt and anger, which cause our high blood pressure, our insomnia and nightmares, which lead to our miserable distress. People who are loving and forgiving are peaceful and genuinely happy.

5. <u>Learn to relax and have fun.</u> After God created the world, He rested on the 7th day. When we take time to relax for even 15 minutes from work each day, we become more productive and we're easy to get along with.

6. <u>It pays to be knowledgeable</u>. Find time to read inspirational books that are beneficial to your spiritual, physical, and mental health such as the Holy Bible and other soul up-lifting literatures.

7. <u>Take responsibility for your happiness.</u> It is said

that happiness is our own making. Here is a sound saying: "In order to multiply happiness, one should divide it with others."

8. <u>Adopt a prudent philosophy in life.</u> This will give you meaning and direction such valuable convictions as: respecting the rights of others; helping people in time of need; and leading a well-balanced lifestyle.

9. <u>Count your blessings and be thankful</u>. We should always thank the Lord for all the blessings we received and protecting us from evil. The only things God wants from us is gratefulness.

10. <u>Always feel God's presence amidst us</u>. As faithful God's children, let us never forget for a moment that: "When two or more are gathered together in Jesus' name, there I AM in their midst." God's help is only a prayer away.

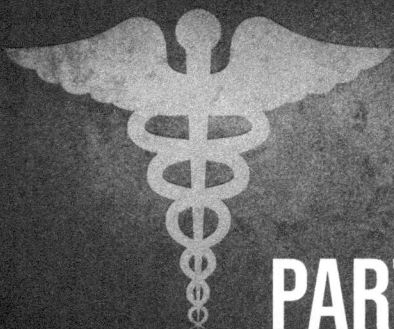

PART VIII

PHOBIAS, VIOLENCE AND SUFFERINGS

Phobia-Irrational Fear

*"Some men are mad if
they behold a cat."*
William Shakespeare

All of us has a share of phobia towards animals, insects and some situations. Nobody is spared from fear of any kind. Of course, there are realistic or normal universal fears like experiencing an earthquake, tsunami, facing a hungry lion and other ferocious man-eating animals. Most people are not afraid of domesticated animals like dogs (unless they are mad dogs) and cats.

If fear is slight, then it doesn't bother at all. However, when the fear is in a discernable degree that it interferes and adversely affect our lives, then that is something strange. Surprisingly, even Brad Pitt, the famous masculine Hollywood star, is terribly afraid of sharks; Steven Spielberg fears reptiles (zoophobia). Other well-known world personalities like Howard Hughes, the American airplane tycoon is fearful of germs (mysophobia). Former President Ronald Reagan dreads flying during his acting career (aerophobia). Even Sigmund Freud, the father of modem psychoanalysis, suffered from "cardiac neurosis" (Thanatophobia or fear of death).

Nowadays, some people here is Dumaguete and anywhere are fearful of the thought of leaving the safety of their house and becomes agarophobic as well as pyrophobic (fear of fire). They feel insecure for some reasons: presence of hired killers, robbers, thieves and even helpers with hairy hands, for they might steal their belongings.

Phobia is defined as an unreasonable fear. It is an irrational fear of a particular object or situation. Once the phobia is fully developed, the individual will do anything in his power to avoid coming into contact with the feared object or situation, or anything that has become strongly associated with that object or situation. This is known as "Phobic /disorder" in psychiatry.

When the individual restricts the freedom of his action and as long as he avoids and focuses on the source of his phobia, he remains relatively comfortable. The symptom varies from mild uneasiness to panic reaction. Symptoms include: fast heartbeat, sweating, tremors, lump in the throat, stomach cramps, shortness of breath, sense of impending deem or death and overwhelming need to flee-"I've got to get out of here quickly."

There are over 500 phobias listed, but the common ones are:

Simple phobia-involves fear of animals or some objects
Social phobia-fear of being scrutinized by others
Agoraphobia-fear of leaving home or open spaces

Aculophobia–– fear of the dark
Acrophobia-fear of heights
Algophobia-fear of pain
Aquaphobia-fear of water
Astrophobia-fear of lightning
Brontophobia-fear of thunder
Cynophobia- fear of dogs
Cancerophobia-fear of cancer
Mysophobia- fear of germs
Pyrophobia-fear of fire
Thanatophobia–– fear of death
Triskaidekaphobia-fear of the No. 13
Xenophobia-fear of strangers
Zoophobia–– fear of animals

Social Phobia

(The title means "fear of people.")

Filipinos are generally known to be shy people or *mahiyain,* except for those who have been exposed to other Western culture and have been influenced by such foreign culture, so much so that they become very sociable, very vocal, and very demonstrative in their way of life.

It cannot be denied that in a typical, conservative Filipino home, children are never allowed to answer back nor reason out their parents when reprimanded. When there are visitors in the house children should stay away from the visitors and keep themselves in the room quietly. They could come out when visitors are done and gone.

The lifestyle or training of children at home are carried or identified even when they are already in school. The teacher could identify the kind of family each child belongs to according to his attitude and behavior towards his classmates in the class and towards his teacher.

It is very pathetic and too tragic for a parent to learn from school that one of his children is suffering from extreme shyness. He does not participate in any class activity. He becomes nervous and tongue-tied whenever he is called upon to recite. He becomes very anxious and manifests tremors or feels in cold sweat. His close make friend would notice that he could not urinate in the presence of others. He seems to be a loner. Much more he could not eat with other people, except with his own immediate family.

Cause: A very traumatic childhood history. This guy knows that there is something wrong in him but he can't help it.

Management: Psychotherapy is highly recommended!

Triskaidekaphobia-Fear of No. 13

"Nothing is either good or bad,
but thinking makes it so."
William Shakespeare

Undoubtedly, countless people in the world have morbid fear towards the No. 13, more so if it falls on a Friday. Nobody wants to be number 13. Why is this so?

Let us unravel some reasons why people associate number 13 as an unlucky number. Practically, all people in the whole world have been subjected to unfound tales of folklores and mythology, repeatedly told to them by imaginative parents and guardians during sleeping time. On top of this, it is reinforced by the disciplinary admonitions by injecting fear such as threats of punishments (physical and verbal) with the aim of controlling their negative impulses or drives. This will consequently result to negative belief, a start of a phobic reaction. Children are suggestible and gullible. For instance, when the parents would tell a son or daughter not to go out at night for it is a 13th day and a Friday at that. The date and day are believed too risky and unlucky. This parental warning becomes a negative stimulus to the deep psyche of the child. This becomes an unresolved conflict and thus disturbs the troubled mind of the affected child. Hence, the conflict mind becomes accident-prone and thus the self-fulfilling prophecy is fulfilled.

There are a number of theories why number 13 is connoted as an unlucky number. In numerology, the No. 13 is believed to be a number of completeness. In history, the Knights Templar is arrested on the 13th day and a Friday. The "Ides of March" is believed to fall on a 13. Sociologists discover that most accidents that kill most victims fall on a Friday, the 13th. But the theory that explains why the No. 13 is unlucky is only in the mind of the believer.

What is Fear?

"Fear always springs from ignorance."
Emerson, the American Scholar

Our creator has infuse emotion as part of our human nature and programmed into all the animals and people so as to instinctually response to potential danger.

What is fear? Biologically speaking, when a person

experiences fear, certain areas in his brain such as the **amygdala** and the **hypothalamus** are immediately activated and appear in control, the first response to fear. Chemicals such as **adrenaline** and the stress hormone **cortisol** are released into the blood stream causing certain physical reaction such as: rapid heartbeat, increase blood pressure, tightening of muscles, sharpened or redirected senses, and dilatation of the pupils (to let in more light), increase sweating.

People who experienced this often remember the moment when disasters struck and how time seemed to slow down. They knew exactly what to do without consciously thinking about it. They had great strength. Some had even able to lift a car, to save their trapped child and they felt no pain. All these are protective mechanism to increase our chances of survival.

Fear is not always adaptive. For instance, a small amount of fear is needed before an important speech serves a purpose-it encourages one to focus on his topic and avoid making a fool of oneself. This is one of the types of fear that can be useful to sharpen our mind. However, some types of fear that are excessive can become crippling. Psychiatrists call these kinds of fear as **phobia.** There are several kinds of phobia. The following are irrational or morbid kinds of fear. For example, fear of strangers is called **xenophobia;** fear of hair is **chaetephobia;** fear of flying is **aviophobia;** fear of confined space is **claustrophobia;** fear of paper is **payrophobia**. (For more, see page 232.)

Future-oriented fear is **anxiety.** We don't know what's going to happen next and we cannot control upcoming events.

Management: Your holistic Psychiatrist can help permanently resolve your fear. Consult him.

Anxiety and Fear Control

"Fear always springs from ignorance."
Emerson

Definitely, emotion plays an important role in our daily lives. Anxiety and fear are such essential emotions that are basically programmed into the brain as an instinctual response to potential danger that may arise in this world.

Anxiety is the internal anticipatory feeling of dread, apprehension and impending danger or catastrophe. It is a future-oriented fear. And fear the danger is external and directly perceived and the source is largely or wholly perceived. When one is actually confronted with the fearful object, fear and anxiety reactions tend to overlap. The physiological changes are similar. Many situations in life arouse mixed feelings of fear and anxiety. Example: One feels **anxious** when he hears a bad news, but he **fears** a big dog rushing towards him.

Biologically speaking, when a person experiences intense anxiety and fear, neurologists claim that certain areas in the brain such as **amydala** and the **hypothalamus** are immediately activated and control the physical responses to fear. Neurotransmitters or chemicals such as **adrenaline** and the stress hormone **cortisol** are released into the bloodstream causing physical symptoms such as: *Rapid heartbeat, Increase blood pressure, Tension or tightening of muscles, Sweating or cold clammy perspiration, Pallor, Headache, Dizziness, Stomach upset, Faintness, Chest pain, Lost of appetite.*

All these are protective mechanisms to increase our chances of survival. Most stable and emotionally mature individuals in life can adequately handle and outgrow their fears. This is normal anxiety. However, there are excessive types of fear that can become crippling and victimize vulnerable individuals we call "neurotics" -unrealistically anxious people. They are apt to suffer from "phobic disorders". Phobia is an unrealistic morbid fear of object or situation. This is abnormal anxiety.

Principles of Management:

Psychiatrists advocate Cognitive Therapy and Behavior Modification; Technique Therapy for Severe Phobic Disorders. For less severe Anxiety Disorders, try any of the following:

- Breathing Therapy (slow and deep breathing)
- Learn a Relaxation Technique; aerobics, walking, jogging, swimming, cycling
- Listening to melodious music
- Meditation-Prayer and spiritual therapy has all calming effects.

Causes of Criminality

*"Society prepares for crime,
the criminal commits it."*

Buckle

Every law-abiding citizen in this "City of Gentile People" (Dumaguete) is alarmed and concerned on the surge of criminality (particularly on unsolved killings) with no apparent solution at hand. People in this university town are so much affected and are praying for its eventful solution by our duly constituted authorities. Of course, this is a sublime task for everyone-the local government, socio-civic groups, the religious, the academe and not only to rely on the serious and relentless efforts of our PNP in curbing criminality of a growing metropolis.

Researchers have found that there are inevitable factors in life that invariably influence the commission of crimes. And the consistent report is that **Poverty and Anti-Social Behavior** tend to be linked together. Specific causes of criminality on society varies largely. It ranges from chromosomal (XYY) aberration to brain damage due to effects of drugs, alcohol, and physical injuries; extreme deprivations of basic human needs; poor moral and spiritual value formation since childhood and bad juvenile influences; poor parental modeling and identification of sociopathic parents; unemployment; unresolved hostility against authorities; chaotic and amoral environment; extremely materialistic society obsessed with money and wealth; sordid influences of mass media-uncontrolled showing of violence over TV, internet, movie shows, smut and crime in printed and video form, etc. with double-bind messages (good and evil messages), which subtly influence the gullible young minds.

Take for instance the movie, "Catch Me If You Can" where actor Leonardo Dicarpio played the role of a con-man and thief, of which the authorities used him to solve crimes. Perhaps, adults understand this double-edge philosophy-"It needs a thief to catch another thief." The subtle lesson is clear: One can steal/kill without being caught. Some would say this is "smart." Indeed? The Cebuanos termed it as "Pa-abtik Technique" (a fast draw).

In a too materialistic society, money is equated with wealth, power, satisfaction or survival in a highly competitive world. Money becomes the greatest motivator of the world. A deprived, hungry and disgruntled people can possibly do anything-steal, kill, take high risks, enslave themselves, etc. just to have money at any cost. A very frightening principle.

Theologians hold that it is not money per se that is the root of all evil, rather, it is the <u>love of</u> money.

Acceptability, today, many people utterly lack true spirituality and do not fear God anymore. Hence, criminality flourishes in our midst. However, probably, it could be minimized through effective ways instituted by brilliant and God-inspired authorities by truly helping the dire needs of the "Least, the Last, and the Lost" among us. Hopefully, peace, love and harmony could reign once more in our society.

Signs of Insecurities of the Times

At this present time, one can feel and see the apparent manifestations of serious **insecurities** among our people. These obvious reactions must be the direct or indirect results of the various **crimes** people learn from the mass media–– the daily news that are blurted from the different radio and TV stations and gossips from people.

The unmistaken and tangible signs of insecurities that one can observe among the people in the city are:

1. They have their cars' windshield tinted very dark tints (black) that one could hardly see the driver or passenger. (These are authorities who have lots of enemies.)
2. Unsecured individuals have their concrete walls built so high that robbers could hardly climb them.

3. They put broken glasses (shards) on top of the walls around their houses.
4. They buy expensive watchdogs to guard their house against the thieves.
5. They hire security guards to watch not only their commercial buildings but also their houses against burglars.
6. They install a sensitive electric gadget that lights when a person passes by.
7. They buy hand pistols and licensed high power rifles to use against intruders.
8. Now is the latest CCTV (Closed Circuit Television) of which the owner installs in strategic corners of their house to focus and record any activity or event of the day.
9. But the most dangerous device is the installation of a high voltage tension wire around the fence to electrocute burglars when they try to enter the house (this can be very dangerous to members of your own families... **never do this!).**

Violence--An Evil Act of Man

Violence is a very dangerous instrument for it can destroy those who wield it."
John Gardner

Undoubtedly, the whole world has focused its utter attention to the recent barbaric act of violence committed by power-hungry politicians in brutally murdering 64 innocent civilians including 27 journalists (mostly women) in the Maguindanao mass carnage.

Let us then try to understand the psychology of

violence. Psychologists simply describe violence as an act of aggression. Aggression is defined as a behavior intended to injure another person who does not want to be injured.

As a psychiatrist, I can truly attest that most violent individuals in our society, as people see, are not mentally ill per se (or frankly psychotic) or clearly definable as patients and therefore, they are best handled by legal authorities. Most psychiatrists usually avoid managing personality-disordered individuals.

In psychiatric emergency, patients who are diagnosed as major psychiatric disorders that may present violent behaviors include those who are truly suffering from schizophrenia, organic brain disorder, substance abuse, alcoholism, dementia, seizure (epileptic) disorder and other unclassified types. All these patients show short-term risks of violence due to either organic (physical) or chemical changes in the brain, which cause impaired impulse control and hence, the uncontrollable violent outbursts.

However, the real culprit (pathology) of most criminal behavior who unreasonably commit heinous crimes, such as rape, murder in cold blood, etc. are termed in psychiatry as Anti-Social Personality Disorder, also referred to as sociopath. This particular person is living normally among other persons in the community who appears (camouflage) as a "wolf in sheep's clothing." It is difficult to identify him outright.

A well-known sociopath in history was the Oklahoma Bomber Timothy McVeigh, a US Green Beret Sgt. And a Desert Storm veteran. His only conflict was he "hated the American government." So, he planned and mercilessly detonated his bomb-laden van besides a government building, killing scores of people in it, including school children.

Definitely, there is now an awesome world indignation condemning this extremely barbaric act of mass murder in Maguindanao. We can say that this heinous and ruthless massacre is a timely wake-up call to all our lawmakers of our country. There is a dire need for our Congress and Senate to legislate stringent laws to finally stop and dismantle political dynasties, warlordism, private militia and other abuses that will continue to victimize our helpless citizens. Certainly, this slaughter of the innocents is a triumph of Satanism in our civilized and Christian society, which strongly advocate love and peace. What an irony indeed!

The Root Causes of Violent Aggression

*"To everything there is a season and a
time to every purpose under heaven.
A time to kill and a time to heal..."*
Ecclesiastes 30:3, KJV

The gruesome shooting of 20 children (ages 6 to 7) and 7 adults (including his own mother whom he shot earlier in their house) at Sandy Hook Elementary School, Newtown, Connecticut, U.S.A. by a 20-year old untreated autistic kid last December 28, 2012, was a classical example of an extremely violent aggression. Alan Lanza used an automatic assault rifle and two automatic pistols owned by his mother in gunning down the 27 innocent people.

There were a number of school campus shootings before in the U.S. although the killers shot themselves when the police cornered them.

America is a too permissive country in owning a gun. Americans have a favorite motto: "Have gun, will travel." It's easy to purchase a gun or two for family's protection in the U.S. There are so many untreated neurotics and agitated depressed multiracial and prejudiced individuals walking around in the streets who can kill anytime. Americans and other races are extremely under stressed and are potentially homicidal.

Psychiatrists define aggressive behavior as any act that is intended to do physical or psychological harm.

Behavioral experts discuss the potential causes that contribute to violent aggression in man:

1. Hereditary (Genetic)-Criminally-inclined family with XXY chromosomes. Example: Speck killed a number of American and Filipino nurses in the U.S.
2. <u>Personality influenced by environmental factors. Exposure to violence in the neighborhood.</u>
3. Excess of serotine in the brain triggers violence (Research finding.)
4. Exposure to a traumatic family background; constant quarrels; fighting, etc; severe punishment by cruel parents.
5. Children who are frequently expose to various violent TV and movie shows can unconsciously imbibe the evil lessons.
6. Unresolved hostility and revenge towards a person or group of people. Example: Hitler hated and killed millions of Jews.
7. The innate search and craving of protein for food. Example: A Gorilla kills another chimpanzee for its protein need.
8. Paranoid Schizophrenic can kill himself

following his auditory hallucination-"kill yourself."

9. An agitated depressed person can be so hostile and may run amok and kills himself.

All the above negative behaviors can push a person to be violently aggressive.

The Alarming Increase of Domestic Violence (Wife Beating)

When love turns to hate, "Hell hath no fury like a woman scorned."
William Congreve

We often read in the newspapers of wives or girlfriends being beaten up by their husbands or boyfriends. Domestic violence or also called "<u>Battered Wife Syndrome</u>" is a very significant social and legal issue in our society. It is also known as medico-legal issue for it involves both medical (health) and legal (law) problems. Most often psychiatrists are called upon to handle the victim for it adversely affects treatable primarily <u>psyche</u> (mind) and not only the physical aspect, which is easily treatable.

The prevalence of domestic violence in the U.S. varies. But it is estimated to be 2 to 4 million women every year are believed to be victimized. We do not have an exact number of Filipinos who are victimized by domestic violence but noticeably, the news reports are alarming. It is believed that domestic violence is the most common cause of traumatic injury to women.

Domestic or sometimes called "partner violence" involves actual use of physical force or threat by a spouse, sexual abuse, psychological abuse, economic control, and progressive social isolation. This occurs whether the abuser is angry, drunk, or even in a calm state. Some men suffer psychological abuse, too, by dominated wives. The abuser partner may have been abused or witnessed abuse while growing up as studies revealed.

Physical abuse may be preceded or accompanied by emotional abuse. A wife may be emotionally abused is she is regularly insulted and made to feel worthless-i.e. such derogatory remarks as *"Wala kang hiya, wala kay nahot o kapuslanan nga asawa ka,"* (You are shameful, you are a worthless wife!) or any other humiliating or threatening remarks from the husband. The wife is always placed in a constant fear. These helpless women are repeatedly beaten by their husbands who are being kept secret from being known in public.

Women should know that the abuse may get worse especially in this stressful time and may even end in death of the victims. Every woman must know that no one has the right to injure you. <u>Violence is definitely against the law.</u>

Victims should report all attacks or beating to the authorities (police). <u>Blotter all injuries to document the abuse</u>. Tell confidently to somebody you trust (your doctor, spiritual adviser, a close friend or family member) in what happened to you. It is also important to have a safety plan in case you are threatened. Planning ahead may help you what to do in the future. Keep a telephone <u>number</u> of any person or agency (PNP, Crisis Center, etc.) and call those when you need help. There is now a law against women abusers. Don't be afraid to report any <u>abuser.</u> It's your prerogative, woman. Do it!

Remember, <u>no one wants to live with a cruel person,</u>

unless one is a masochist (a person who loves to receive PAIN).

The Significance of PAIN in our Life

During the Lenten Season, the whole of Christendom is timely reminded of the most painful Passion of our Lord Jesus Christ who suffered the most ignominious death of crucifixion to redeem us from our sins. Historians attested that the crucifixion is the most brutal and cruel form of death ever imposed on mankind.

It cannot be denied that man, from birth to death, has experienced the feeling of pain from minor to major forms; so much so that man is able to deal with the chronic or long-term suffering--whether physical, emotional or spiritual pain.

There are people who can cope with the minor injuries in their lives; such fleeting pains like headaches, toothaches and other slight injuries. But some individuals are unfortunate that they have to suffer the major and very serious painful injuries in life like fractures, the major illness like cancers, etc. Fortunately scientists discovered a natural painkiller in our body known as **endorphins.** This substance relieves any severe pains felt in the body.

Doctors define pain as an unpleasant or an uncomfortable sensation that ranges from mild irritation to excruciating agony. It is the most commonly reported symptom and is linked with enumerable disorders and diseases. It is a clue in diagnosis. It is most commonly a symptom of disease, injury, or abnormal changes in the body. For instance, if the pain is constantly found at the right lower quadrant of the abdomen and it becomes tender (painful) upon palpitation, then the doctor would say, "It is appendicitis." When the pain is felt away from the organ, it is referred to as **referred pain.** A sign of heart ailment is usually felt with a pain radiating to the left arm towards the left middle and ring finger.

When one is in pain due to injury or illness, it stops him from his work and it means that he has to rest. If the pain persists and is becoming worse, despite his own home-treatment, he is forced to seek treatment by consulting a doctor for proper management. Early pain is a timely signal by the Almighty God to save us from the worse consequences in life. Always remember the great saying: "No pain, no gain."

Always pray to be able to bear or cope with the pain "our cross" God gives us to carry in our life. St. Thomas More implicitly said: "Earth has no sorrow that Heaven cannot heal."

Traumatic Experiences of Life

"Adversity reveals genius,
prosperity conceals it."

Horace

One way or another, everyone has underwent unpleasant experiences in life since birth. No one is spared from any painful episode for this is a normal part of living. "No pain, no gain," as the saying goes.

Doctors define trauma as a wound or injury, either physical or psychological. Psychological traumas are deeply disturbing experiences, which produce overt or repressed emotional reactions and render the individual vulnerable to later stresses.

Karen Horney, a Neo-Freudian psychoanalyst, holds that early traumatic experiences produces "weak spots" in the human psychological armor, which may later become the nucleus for neurotic reactions. Psychiatrists found that a large number of schizophrenics (persons with severe mental disorder) has suffered extreme traumatic events in their lives.

Examples of traumatic experiences in childhood are: lack of mothering as in early death of a mother, parental rejection, early separation of parents, school failures, social rejection, etc.

Traumatic episodes in adulthood are total failure in marriage, job demotion or loss, discrimination, stressful situations such as floods, earthquakes, war, etc.

Neurosurgeons and trauma specialists report major physical traumatic episodes such as blows or injuries to the head that produce acute or chronic brain disorder. More severe brain injuries may result in the loss of intellectual functions. In psychiatry, there is post-traumatic stress disorder (PTSD) where people have undergone overwhelming stresses in their lives. These individuals became psychologically and mentally crippled. Without the benefit of a long and intensive psychotherapy, they suffer constant fear, always intense and anxious, withdrawn, unable to sleep and never enjoy any happiness in their lives anymore. Most are depressed and many have committed suicide because of severe depression.

After an extreme emotional trauma, psychiatrist and clinical psychologists have a special tool in managing the victim through an effective psychological process called "critical debriefing." This maneuver is used to help the victim become normal again by readjusting to adverse situations in life.

As Christians, we were taught that the road in this world is not always "strewn with flowers." Jesus says,

"In this world you will have tribulations but be of good cheer. I have overcome the world." (John 16:33, KJV). Chiara Lubich taught us in the Focolare movement that everyone has his own forsakenness as Jesus cried out while He was being crucified. "My God, My God, why hast thou forsaken me?"

In spite all the traumatic experiences in life we should never give up hope. Because even in the darkest moments of our lives, hope can pull us through a trauma. As Psalm 41 states, "The Lord will deliver me in times of troubles." Have always a strong faith my friends.

The Mystery of Suffering

> *"The sufferings of the present times are not worthy to be compared with the glory which will be revealed to us."*
> Romans 8:18, KJV

The sages say that suffering is part and parcel of human existence. People always associate suffering with painful living, and the psychologist connects it to stressful conditions. From birth to death, every living creature experiences suffering in one way or another. For instance, some suffer physical pain-like infections, heart attack, stroke, kidney failure, cancer, accidents, etc, while others suffer from mental or emotional sufferings-such as loss or death of love ones, nervous breakdown, etc., or financial sufferings-like bankruptcy, unemployment or loss of job, poverty; natural disasters-such as typhoons, floods, epidemics, conflagration, etc.

When we were born, the very person who primarily experienced the most painful suffering of labor was our mother. But her intimate ordeal of motherhood is tangibly rewarded with a smiling bundle of joy!

In the Old Testament, the common belief of ancient people is that the Almighty God gives punishment to the disobedient people in the form of sufferings-such as floods, lightning, afflictions, invalidism, etc. However, He sometimes gives or allows severe afflictions even to righteous people as exemplified in the Story of Job in the Holy Bible. When God gives a person a trial, given test of suffering, He is also ready to reward him just what He did to Job, as well as to the saints, and to other repentant sinners.

Here is a meaningful quotation from St. Thomas More: **"Earth has no sorrow that Heaven cannot heal."** The lesson is clear-a faithful who always dedicates his sorrows or sufferings to the Lord has a great chance to go to Heaven.

When I was a young man, I read St. Thomas Akimpes' **book-"Imitation of Christ."** The book suggested that we should give all our sufferings, pains, and forsakenness to Jesus Christ who suffered and died for us on the cross.

The Value of Suffering

"There can be no real and abiding
happiness without sacrifice."
H. W. Sylvester

The whole of Christendom celebrates Holy Week, a very solemn time for all faithful to offer sacrifices and repentance for their sinful ways.

Historically, the people of Nineveh were spared by God from destruction when they repented by wearing sackcloth and ashes (Gospel). This is a clear indication that God would want all of us to atone for our sins. However, there are people in our society who hide behind the false mask and deny their sufferings and pretend they are not there. The result is loneliness and hypocrisy. For proud and hostile people who like some individuals to suffer because of their vindictive attitude, they will also doubly suffer for their evil deeds and intentions. These double-faced persons who appear to be friendly outside but actually want to destroy you by ridiculing, criticizing and outing you down to shame are known as "modem Pharisees"-the real hypocrites. A good spiritual advice from a holy person: "Be silent in the face of false accusation. Show love to a friend who betrays you and do not retaliate for these are the opportunities for self-sacrifice and sanctification.

Cardinal Richard Cushing of Boston, U.S.A. has a beautiful Morning Prayer that touches on suffering. He prays: "My dearest Lord, what do you send me today? Humiliations, contradictions, physical sufferings, bad news which I do not expect, an aching heart, a failure? Shall I see myself misjudged, insulted, wrongly suspected, and despised? If I am discouraged, raise me up. But through it all teach me to say, 'THY WILL BE DONE' Amen."

There are still people in this world whose characters and basic human attitudes are pillars of strength and steadfastness despite all the miseries of life. These are the people who are solid in their faith. They know the true value of suffering that cleans, heals and brings love, peace and joy. To quote the Vietnamese Archbishop Nguyen Van Tuan: "Sacrifice is the true proof of love." This has been exemplified by the greatest and ultimate suffering of Jesus Christ on the Cross-a Redeeming Love of All.

Remember: "If you expect to avoid suffering, then, do not expect to become a saint." (A holy person.)

Types of Disaster Victims

"Suffering is part and parcel of human existence–– a problem not to be solved, but mystery to be lived."
Fr. Bel San Luis

Every human being must always be ready for the unexpected natural adverse phenomenon or terrible disaster that may occur anytime in life. The traumatic events that are described to be outside the range of common human experience are bereavement, chronic illness, or loss of job.

Typhoon "Yolanda" the extra-ordinary natural disaster terribly devastated Leyte, Samar, Northern part of Cebu and other Eastern Visayas region, so much so that it resulted to the death of a number of people and the destruction of homes, commercial buildings, hospitals, workplaces, farms and other vital properties. But worse is the "Post-Traumatic Stress Disorder" (PTSD) that is being suffered and experienced by the typhoon victims because of the extreme deprivation of the human dire needs such as food, water, shelter, clothing, medicines, electric energy and other life-sustaining elements.

Studies have shown that a strong disaster will produce four (4) types of victims (Survivors):

1. The Severely Injured. These patients direly need immediate help or attention to their physical and mental injuries. They become a nervous wreck.

2. The Uninjured Survivors. They suffer mental shock, guilt feelings, helplessness, insecurity, utter frustration, discouragement and nervousness.
3. Relative of Victims. They also suffer feelings of guilt, helplessness, misgivings, insecurity, depression, anger and discouragement.
4. Disaster Workers. They are also psychologically affected. They suffer insomnia, nightmares, anxiety, depression and nervousness.

Management:

They need crisis intervention or mental debridement to desensitize them from the psychic trauma. The general aim of this therapeutic essential process is to help the person of family make the best use of available resources in the environment and facilitate further treatment needed to achieve and complete the healing process of mental, physical and spiritual stability of the victim in order to be normal again. This is a must.

For the non-victims, always thank the Almighty God for sparing us from the severe calamities in life.

Portrait of an Abuser (A Fake Lover)

*"An abuser is the real wolf
in sheep's clothing."*

Anonymous

Today, people often hear or read in the newspapers the derogatory word "abuse" such as "drug abuse, physical abuse, verbal abuse, sexual abuse, etc." This term is also synonymous to "domestic violence or battered wife/

child." This significant social problem is indiscriminately committed mostly by cruel and sadistic men with personality defect. They victimize their too compliant or inadequate wife who just endured the miserable relationship because she is afraid to lose her husband or fear of being killed by him. Other victims of abuse are children and other subordinates.

As an experienced Expert Court Witness in the annulment of loveless marriages, I have to prove that the abuser has seriously transgressed the Family Code of the Philippines before the Honorable Judge will hand down the verdict of legal separation.

Authorities define abuse as "any treatment that negatively impacts and transgresses the rights and the self-worth of another person."

Statistics show that roughly 60% of men who batter their wives are said to be angry and want to gain power by humiliating them. Authorities said that after all, sexual abuse is not really about sex, but it is about dominance and control. The rapist is identified as the foremost mean abuser known to man.

The characteristic traits of Abuser Persons are:

1. They were likely to have been abused by either parent during childhood or adolescence.
2. Emotionally unstable or immature persons.
3. They are intolerant or hostile towards life in general.
4. Show little or no remorse of conscience.
5. Put the blame for one's mistakes on the other person.
6. Cynical, judgmental, and unable to trust people.
7. Low self-esteem, lacks social skills.
8. Rationalize and deny abuse (pathological lying).

9. Very defensive when angered.
10. Use power and control to gain advantage in relationships.
11. Use shame and guilt to manipulate others and may threaten suicide if spouse attempts to leave or end relationship.
12. A manipulative and appears to be a nice or charming guy outwardly.
13. Do not allow the other person to articulate her feelings.
14. Withhold financial resources.
15. Verbally or physically humiliate the other person through inappropriate gestures, comments or jokes, plus other negative traits.

The typical abuser is a "sociopath" (Antisocial Personality Disorder) who apparently appears charming or "guapo" (handsome) but in reality, he is a downright dangerous guy, who can potentially kill his spouse through mental and physical torture. A message of concern to all the decent women. Be sure to marry a man with proven Sterling Character but never, never an "ABUSER!" Regrets always come last...right?

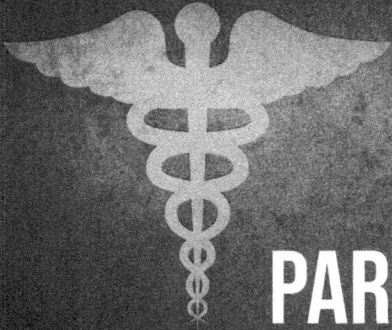

PART IX

THE VALUE OF BEING ACTIVE AND FIT

The Importance of Exercise and Being Fit

To have an improved quality life it is important to be being active and fit. Research shows that fitness is a strong measure of health. In a study of more than 25,000 volunteers, researchers found that a person's fitness level was more important than body weight. Men in the study who were overweight or obese but who were physically fir had a lower risk of death than men who were a healthy weight but were not physically fit. Being fit improves your overall health and reduces your rick of disease.

Let's enumerate the benefits and divide it into the following terms.

Short-Term Benefits:

- A healthier heart. Physical activity makes demands on your heart that make it stronger and better able to function.
- Healthy muscles, bones and joints. Resistance training such as weight lifting improves

muscular strength and endurance and increases bone density, which is especially important for older adults to prevent falls and injuries.

- Increased burning of calories. Physical activity burns calories and helps you achieve a healthy balance between the calories you take in from food and those you expend. When you exercise regularly, your body burns more calories, both during activity and at rest. Being fit may also lower your percentage of body fat and increase muscle strength and tone. Your percentage of body fat depends on genetics, lifestyle, and physical activities. No matter what your size or shape, physical activity has important health benefits, including-
  A. Better ability to cope with stress. People who are fit have less anxiety, depression, and stress than people who aren't active.
  B. Improved ability to fall asleep and sleep well.
  C. Increased energy.
  D. Increase mental acuity, sharper and faster thinking.

Long-Term Benefits:

- Reduce the risk to die early.
- Reduce of developing coronary artery disease. Mean who are not active have about twice the risk of developing heart disease than men who are regularly physically active.
- People who get regular physical activity as part of a cardiac rehabilitation program have a lower risk of dying from a heart attack.

- Regular physical activity can also lower blood pressure in those who have high blood pressure.
- Physical activity may prevent type 2 diabetes through its effect on insulin, how the body processes sugar, and maintenance of body weight.
- Reduce the risk of developing colon and other cancers.
- Have a lower risk to become obese.

But please bear in mind that for most people, they should talk to a health professional first before beginning a regular exercise program, especially those who have conditions such as coronary artery disease, high blood pressure, heart valve disease, or diabetes. If you are at risk for or have some of these conditions, your health professional may want to help you build a plan matched to your needs. He or she may want to do tests before you start a plan or want you to be more careful and watch for injuries or other problems.

The Greatest Benefits of Exercise

"Take regular exercise. Exercise strengthens your heart, improves blood Circulation, loosens up your joints, energizes and aerates your lungs."

Frederick Stare

Physiologists say that an organ that is used is bound to deteriorate. It only develops when it is properly used. The human body has more than 500 muscles. To keep these muscles strong, a person must exercise regularly.

Our muscles work with the rest of our body to make us move and alive. By exercising regularly our body learns to pump enough oxygen to our muscles and other vital organs.

How do we keep ourselves look great? Doing exercise is the best way to achieve this. It pumps blood and the needed oxygen to all parts of the body. This makes us feel alert, active and happy. Exercise definitely makes our muscles firm and strong.

A good exercise program must be done in moderately intensive activity at 3 to 5 times a week of about 15 to 30 minutes.

Nutrition is also important in keeping the muscles healthy. Protein foods such as lean meat, fish and protein supplements help muscles grow. The have the job of building body tissues. Carbohydrates give muscles the energy they need to contract. Carbohydrates are the "fuel" foods. Whole grain and enriched bread, fresh fruits and vegetables have a lot of carbohydrates in them. It is also important to have our blood sugar down as well as the bad saturated fats. We have to drink up to 12 or more glasses of water and organic fruit and vegetable juices daily. Multivitamins such as B-complex, Vitamins C, E and traces of minerals are also needed.

Two highly recommended exercises are:

1. **Aerobic Exercise or Cardiovascular Exercise.** This exercise improves both the respiratory (lungs) and circulatory systems (heart and vessels). Example: Walking, jogging, swimming, cycling.
2. **Resistance Training or Strength-building Exercise.** This increases muscle bulk and strength. Example: Weightlifting.

The benefits of consistent exercise are:

- You lose weight effectively.
- You appear younger and maintain a good figure.
- Less vulnerable to any illness.
- It helps buffer stress.
- It helps release *endorphins--the* happy hormone.
- It increases your life span.

Make your moves and don't be a coach potato.

The Value of Play

> *"Life must be lived as play."*
>
> Plato

Childhood is generally known as "Play Age". Child psychologists describe this particular stage as the "psycho-motor" developmental period wherein the child id observed to be constantly moving, e.g. running, jumping, climbing, etc. This is the basic and essential necessity of growth-the satisfaction of the child's physical need. The common adage which says, "All work and no play makes Juan a dull boy" is really true. It also makes him tense, rigid, timid, and an inflexible person.

The dictionary defines play as any wholesome activity, which is freely sought and pursued for the sake of enjoyment. Play is an instinctual behavior, which is as natural as the drive to eat and sleep needed for growth. Play can benefit the child physically by exercising his muscles, releasing surplus energy, giving him the mastery in coordination, balance, dexterity, endurance and strength.

Play can also cultivate the child's mental capability by stimulating his imagination by challenging him to use his skills and ingenuity in solving problems. Play, as a recreational activity, can develop his social capabilities through give and take, cooperation and respect for rules. Play can also develop his moral values by following thru les and standards of the group and the need for fairness, honesty, self-control, teamwork and sportsmanship. It can help the growing child maintain his psychological balance by a sound outlet for tensions, frustrations as well as acting-out his anxieties, fears, and resentments as well as by verbalizations. And finally, play can give the child a chance to discover and test his interests, needs and abilities. Therefore, he can learn more about his inner potentials.

Today, Child Therapists use "Play Therapy" as their effective device in the treatment of disturbed children. Parents who are very strict or unreasonably over-controlling towards their children and prevent them a chance to play will consequently result in an unstable, unhappy, anxious and timid children. Some may even become mentally ill or psychotic.

Hence, every good parent should realize the ultimate value of play in the growth and development of strong and healthy children.

Dance--a good therapy for all!

> "...And now my heart with pleasure
> fill dances with the daffodils."
> Alfred Tennyson

Filipinos are not only renowned for their singing ability but also excel in the art of dancing. We see the different Festival Dance Groups with their unique and colorful costumes coming from different towns, cities and provinces of the country. Such culturally-motivated and meaningful dances like the "Sinulog of Cebu," "Dinagyang of Iloilo," the "Maskara" of Bacolod, our "Buglasan Festival" and many other festivals are held annually to attract tourists. The latest "Dance Sport," a highly skillful and precise kind of dances like rhumba, cha-cha, tango, waltz, boggie, jive, etc. delivered by Filipino dance experts who have already won prizes in international competitions. We are still developing the highest form of sophisticated dance--the Ballet. There are still few Filipina Ballerinas who have gained world fame on this type of dramatic dance. In the early 60s, our famous "Bayanihan Dance Troupe" had won first place in group dancing abroad.

When I was in my teens, I would never forget the famous Hollywood superb dancers like Fred Astait, Gene Kelly, Cyd Charisse, etc. who captivated the world their marvelous dances.

Now, we see and appreciate the fast steps and agility of our young dancers with their acrobatic dance styles. Many of our middle-age women as well as widows are enjoying Ballroom Dancing escorted with their younger dance instructors. A lot of students frequent the discos on weekends dancing with their friends.

The Encyclopedia cited dance as man's oldest form of art, which reflect his need to communicate his feelings such as joy or grief using his body. Almost all important occasions in the life of primitive man were courtship, marriage, fertility, war, death, worships, etc. even up to this day, youths dance in front of the altar as a form of prayer and praise.

Today, people consider dancing as a form of aerobatic exercise. It is recommended as dance therapy for the elderly not only for their mental well-being but also good for their joints against arthritis as well. Regular dancing could help lose weight by burning a lot of calories and fats as well as achieve a supple and curvaceous body. Many doctors recommend dancing as an aid in strengthening their cardiovascular system thus achieving a healthier heart. Enjoying dancing could ward off stress of daily living and prevent a lot of anxiety and depression.

Economically, professional dancing can definitely augment people's income like these dance instructors and young Filipino women who are trained as dancers for export to countries like Japan, Taiwan, etc. We have now good dancing schools around specializing in ballet lessons, tap dance, even belly dancing and other modern steps to train enthusiasts.

So, let us all cultivate this inherent talent of dancing for the sake of our optimal health of body, mind and spirit. Find time to dance to enjoy life and live longer.

Make Good Reading a Habit

*"Reading is to the mind what
exercise is to the body."*

Addison

Undoubtedly, our early love for reading has greatly helped us formed our basic attitude and values as well as the knowledge and understanding of countless things and happenings in life. We have learned our fundamental knowledge brought about from reading of prescribed textbooks in school and other learning materials from outside. Expert studies have shown that the building of characteristic traits of people are facilitated and largely depend on the lessons and values of what the person had read in his life, which influenced greatly his thinking and lifestyle, like most great men in history experienced.

Let us mention some benefits of reading. Reading, no doubt, enhances our knowledge and the good pleasures of life. It increases our vocabulary and enriches our expressions, expands our understanding of enumerable subjects of interests, brings happiness (i.e. jokes, entertainment, etc), facilitates first-hand information of countless memorable events and happenings in our world as reported in local and national daily newspapers as well as international magazines like Time of Newsweek. The encyclopedia are stacked with interesting data on almost anything found in the universe.

Certainly, reading enhances one's intelligence (IQ), especially one "smartness." One could be a potential "winner" in any contest, be it literary, musical or even political. Consistent reading could make a person to be somebody: like a good teacher, lecturer, speaker or writer, etc. Plus one will never become a "bore" in any friendly company. For sure, you'll be an "entertainer," a "walking dictionary," or a "historian." And much more, nobody will call you an "ignoramus". Believe me.

Most educated and cultured people have been greatly helped in their readings of highly inspiring works of the world's brilliant literary writers, Like Shakespeare, Tolstoy, Destkoevsky, Jules Vemes, Hemingway, of course, every Filipino should read Dr. Jose Rizal's patriotic novels, Noli Me Tangere" and "El Filibusterismo," plus other enumerable books and magazines on almost every subject. As authentic Christians, we don't have to forget to read spiritually-uplifting books like the Holy Bible, Purpose-Driven Life, Good Souls, etc.

Today, there are popular books designed for imaginative youths who eagerly sought the thrills, romance and adventures in life. Series like "Harry Potter: or Ian Fleming's "James Bond series" are examples of good viewing and reading entertainment. Books that twist facts whose authors would try to make it appear as true, should be frowned upon. Those acts are profit-motivated and only determines the mind of the innocent and gullible.

Advice to youths: Aside from reading your schoolbooks, find time in reading other highly educative and informative materials from other books, magazines, etc. Don't depend on internet alone. For as the great writer, Sir Frances Bacon aptly said: "Reading makes a full man." Very true, indeed.

Exercise Your Brain

*"To grow old is the greatest
chapter in the art of living where
real wisdom is fully achieved"*
Oscar Lukefair

Scientific studies by physiologists and educational psychologists have proven that like muscle tissues, the human brain could also be developed in terms of increasing its mental capabilities through a process of "mental calisthenics." American researchers who experimented the brain of animals like chimpanzees and children with average I.Q. have tremendously improved their learning abilities and intellectual performances after subjecting them to a series of mental exercises such as various problems or puzzle solving, spelling difficult words, memorizing poems, and other mental stimulations. Even the average brains of aged people who are not seriously sick with irreversible dementia like Alzheimer's disease could still be helped improve in learning worthwhile activities and prevent rapid mental deterioration.

Many of the well-known personalities in world history accomplished their greatest personal achievements in their advanced age. For instance, the famous satirist, George Bernard Shaw of Britain was 91 years old when he wrote his famous play "Pygmalion," but he lamented. "If only I could live longer to properly benefit from life's experience but regretted that life is wasted on the young." Claude Monet, the French painter was in his 80's when he painted his beautiful "Water Lilies." And Sigmund Freud made valuable writings on psychoanalysis in his 80's. Great Greek philosophers and writers like Plato and Homer have done their works in their old age. And scores of famous men have self-actualized themselves in their "Golden Years."

Here are some effective techniques in exercising and developing the brain:

- Get not a profitable hobby like writing, painting, pet-raising, teaching, etc.
- Play games that challenge your acumen, like cross-word puzzle, chess, card games, mahjongg.
- Try to compose a song, a jingle, a riddle or a joke, etc.
- Increase your vocabulary by learning 5 to 10 new words everyday.
- Do home repairs.
- Memorize a new song, a poem, or a great quotation or passage from the book. Memorize

them well. Recite them when you are taking a bath or exercising.

- Read a selected best seller or a pocket book or any informative piece of literature, i.e. Reader's Digest or spiritual book like the Holy Bible.

If you are really determined to slow down the ravages of aging, then it is so essential to devote a precious time to EXERCISE YOUR GOD GIVEN BRAIN, my friend.

Overcoming the Feeling of Tiredness and Maintaining Energy

Many of us have experienced the lethargic feeling of being tired or fatigue in our life despite a seemingly healthy physical condition. Of course, one naturally gets tired after a long heavy work without rest. However, there are people who apparently have been working regularly like teachers, housekeepers, those other skilled or semi-skilled workers and constantly without complaining of tiredness or fatigue.

There are known causes of tiredness, aside from lack of rest. And it could be due to physical, chemical, or psychological factors that could possibly cause to the monotony and boredom of work. But the major cause of feeling always tired and lack of pep in life is **depression.** This emotional feeling could be caused by any traumatic experience like loss of love object, or death of a love one, loss of job, loss of precious possessions, etc.

The main management of any loss or vim, vigor and vitality, or always feeling tired will depend on the cause.

Here are some suggestions by authorities on how to overcome feelings to maintain energy:

1. Through your thought and faith, keep attached to God, the source of all energy.
2. Avoid the Grey Sickness: half-awake, half-asleep, half-alive, half-dead.
3. Realize that energy sags, when your thoughts sag, so vigilantly keep your thinking alert.
4. Think of yourself as a child of God, a constant recipient of His gifts of boundless health, energy and vitality.
5. Avoid the concept of "growing old and feeble." Picture the youthfulness of your spirit and resisting the aging process.
6. Empty your mind every night as you empty your pocket. Before going to bed, forgive everybody, naming those forgiven. Leave the past in the past, and believe that God watches you as you sleep.
7. Slow down and keep the even rhythm of God
8. Train your mind to block off worry and frustrations, two attitudes which siphon off energy.
9. Affirm that God's constantly renewing energy flows through your being, giving you sufficient vitality to live effectively.

Chemical Factor:

1. Eat fresh fruits rich in potassium and magnesium, like banana and oranges.
2. Take iron pills to prevent anemia that will cause weakness; calcium and sunshine vitamin (Vitamin D) for stronger bones.
3. Exercise for better strength.

Remember the three (3) Rs: **Rest, Relax, Recreate!**

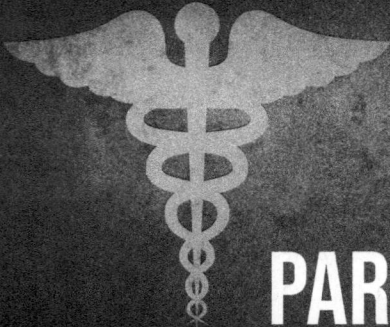

PART X

FACTORS TO CONSIDER IN ACHIEVING SUCCESS

Ambition

*"Ambition should be made
of a sterner stuff"*
William Shakespeare

People always wonder why some persons are so successful in their endeavor in this life and many are not no matter how hard they strive. Of course, nobody could get to be successful by accident. But how do people realize their ambitious pursuit? Does the spark of ambition lie in our genes, family, culture or even in our own hands?

Let us then explore the possible and significant factors that may contribute to the attainment of ultimate success in one's career, business or other precious endeavors in life.

Let us first define what **ambition** means. The Internet defines ambition as the desire for personal achievement. It provides the motivation and determination necessary to achieve a particular end or condition. Ambitious people are characterized by their strong desire for achievement, power, wealth and superiority. For example, the ambition to take advantage of others for personal gain is contemptuous but the ambition to empower others is noble and commendable.

Studies of behaviorists have shown admirable qualities of truly successful people. Generally, ambitious individuals who succeeded in the world such as Dr. Albert Schweitzer of Lamberene, *Africa, who dedicated his whole medical career in treating diseases of poor Africans. Oprah* Windfrey, the famous black American woman, who is an excellent TV hostess and made billions of media empire and many others who started from scraps but now are multi-millionaires.

Their characteristic sterling qualities as a person are: highly integrated persons (loving, kind, honest, simple, humble, helpful); highly goal-oriented; they take high risks; good public relations-"Ambassadors of Goodwill." Tenacity (they persevere to the end); very high self-esteem; and God-fearing. Dr. Daniel Coleman, a behaviorist, writer and lecturer, termed this commendable trait as having a high emotional quotient (E.Q.)-a quality that most charismatic leaders and popular men possess. Let us then strive to be nobly ambitious and not blindly ambitious.

How to Achieve True Success from Failure

According to the Holy Bible, in the Book of Genesis (3:19)- THE FALL OF MAN because of the Sin of Disobedience: God punished Adam by telling him, "By the sweat of your face shall you get bread to eat, until you return to the ground from which you were taken..." God's message is so clear that man has to work in order to live; to work and struggle for survival.

It is tragic to know that there are still some people who believe in bad luck *(dimalas)*. To them there are people who are *bom–– dimalason* (prone to bad luck). This is not true. This is only a gambler's philosophy. The truth is very human being in this world is equally given a chance and opportunity to succeed through his initiative and effort to achieve and fulfill his potentials.

In life, we are always challenged. A determined person will always say, "Either I will find a way, or I will make one." Explorers and inventors always find ways to make people progress and happy. Undoubtedly, we are all inspired by men who are successful after experiencing several discouraging failures in their work. The late Thomas Edison, for example, failed ten thousand times before perfecting the incandescent electric bulb. Otherwise, an average man would have quit at the first failure.

Another inspiring guy is our own Manny Pacquiao. He sadly experienced a number of knockdowns during his early fights. But the humiliating failures never discouraged him. Instead, he continued to have more time for training with a professional and practicing coach until he won The World Boxing Division Records which are hard to break.

Therefore, it is very clear that any genuine success in life could truly be achieved through hard work, with trust in oneself, and most especially trust in God's Divine Mercy.

Be Well Focused

"The unexamined life is not worth living."
Anonymous

The above statement is as true today as it was 23 centuries ago. So let us examine well our life and make up our mind to get it into focus. Everyone knows that if a sight of a gun is not well zeroed to a point, it can never hit the target. This is the *paligaw* (trusting on luck), the trial and error method, which most of the time does not work.

In order to make our life well, orderly and successful, let us first plan well and determine exactly what we want to do. Someone says that it is the clarity of purpose and the intensity of desire, which are the secret ingredients of the magic formula of any success. But this depends largely on the proper factor of motivation, which can greatly contribute to the success of fulfilling any task or occupation in life. Psychologists call this as "achievement motivation".

Nowadays many individuals in our society are successful in their business careers or professions because they are properly trained and well-motivated to improve and innovate on their respective enterprise. Despite setbacks, they don't get discourage so easily and give up. The successful entrepreneurs have a high degree of achievement motivation, which they call, "Accomplishment Feedback"–– a continuous sense of satisfaction in their ability to meet their goals.

There are Filipinos who are highly creative and have a good common sense. What keep them going are: a genuine sense of accomplishment; personal challenges; and words of encouragement. Hence, always focus well in whatever undertaking you venture in life! Most likely you will greatly achieve your goal!

Aptitude--The Measure of Success

Inquisitive people wonder why some persons are successful in their career while others are not. What is the major factor behind why they become truly self-fulfilled in their chosen field of endeavor? Behavioral scientists have found that the single factor and a reliable determinant in the fulfillment of each person's future success is the realization of their personal aptitude in life.

Psychologists define **aptitude** as the likelihood for the future success, usually after motivation and discovery in some given field of endeavor. Aptitude is the predictive measure of a person's likelihood of benefit from motivation or personal experience in a given field; such as art, music, clerical work, mechanical task, or academic studies. Authorities advise parents to observe carefully the individual talent or inclination of each of their children for this true aptitude, and as a good guide for future success and therefore, a fulfillment of their career in life. The problem of most parents is the fact that they tend to dictate their children as to what particular profession they want of them.

Remember that children have their own individual talent and inclination. They want to develop the talent that they have discovered in themselves that they love to do.

Here is a good lesson from an experienced lecturer, that when he was a kid everybody around him noted that he was a very talkative child. When he was in school he manifested his talent in speaking good English. His good grades and remarks in public speaking when he was still a student were his incentives to become a Political Science Graduate major in Public Speaking.

His aptitude paid well when he became a wealthy and famous lecturer and public speaker here and abroad.

Parents, be kind to your children. Don't provoke them to anger!"

Positive Attitude--a Key to Willingness

"The only difference between a good day and a day is one's attitude."
Anonymous

The above paraphrase truly signifies that it's all a matter of choice in whatever we do in this life. One is absolutely free to do whatever he likes of whether it will be for his benefit or suffer the consequence of his action. This is the price of a democratic way of life. Life is a series of experience, trials, and learning opportunities.

Definitely, our success or failure in all these things will greatly depend on our attitude. Our role as human beings is not to be perfect in all the things we do. Our task is to remain resilient. This flexibility is well expressed in the lesson shown by good or clever boxers-"role with the punches". This is a special skill of every boxing technique, which is really hard to hit and difficult to knock down. Of course, you got to have a smart defense, stamina and a power punch to be able to win a fight.

An American holistic physician, Dr. Vernon Sylvester, claims that there is a healthy attitude which is based on faith and healing. This process ultimately boils down to a controlled attitude in responding to life's challenges in ways that honor the sacred nature of our existence. According to the good doctor, God wants us to respond to situations morally, lovingly, and constructively. Our constructive attitude must rid our mind from negative thoughts that are inimical to our human nature.

Definitely, it would be useful to change a negative attitude, which is adversely affecting us. Although changing one's attitude is not easy, psychologists say that attitudes are habits which have been formed slowly since childhood and therefore, it could be changed slowly, too. There are techniques in changing one's attitude of which takes a hard and consistent effort for over a period of months or years.

People with negative attitude are mostly unhappy.

Summarily, our significant attitudes towards wellness are: Respecting the rights of others; sharing what we have; helping people in need; having real friends who are worthy of our trust; having a few books but full of inspiration of greatness; a balance lifestyle; and putting God first in our lives.

The Essence of Decision-making

(See next page)

William Shakespeare, England's greatest dramatist and poet, was right when he- said, "To be or not to be, that is the question." That in life there are many options, and the fulfillment of these desires depends on how one invests on them. All professions are confronted with hard decision-makings.

The factor of decision-making is so essential in whatever undertaking we aspire in life. Most people who experience success in their career or business venture or whatever dealing they are in, it is because of their good decision acumen.

Our daily activity seems to be filled with problems and decision-making. When in crisis decision comes in all sizes big or small, important or trivial ones. At times, we are in great dilemma, and unable to make a good decision. We worry so much if the result of the decision is unfavorable. It takes ample time and energy to arrive at a good decision.

Some factors that help in making a fair and good decision:

- Determine the alternatives
- Study well the problems
- Consult the experienced persons
- Be sure that you are satisfied with your decision

Some Instances:

1. In a family, there is the assurance of the fullest satisfaction of the decision-making in all the vital plans for a family because of the culture that says, "Two heads are better than one," living the Christian way of life with the communion of goods and ideas, and most especially of the love that binds each member of the family.
2. In the hospital, doctors have a difficult time deciding whether or not to pull out the oxygen, for the family could no longer afford to spend the costs of oxygen.
3. In the government, the greatest problem during election is that most people, rich and poor or even the educated ones are easily bribed. Hence, the qualified candidates couldn't win for most of the honest ones don't have enough money to spend.
4. In history, U.S. President Harry Truman was questioned by his Cabinet Members of his plan

to drop the Atomic Bomb in Japan to end the war. His Cabinet Members did not like the idea for fear it would cause the death of millions of innocent civilians---children, young and old. Truman was in a great dilemma. But finally he said that if we won't do this extreme sacrifice, the Japanese Imperial Army would continue to dominate the World and could invade the U.S. Truman finally decided to drop the Atomic Bombs in Hiroshima and Nagasaki, causing the unconditional surrender of Japan, thus ending World War II.

Qualities of a Good Leader

"Leadership is action, not position."
Donald H. Common

Here are valuable traits that constituents mostly desire in a good political Candidate:

- Good Character. A person who absolutely hates dishonesty and corruption; one who is humble and approachable; a well-disciplined person with good "PR" (Public Relations).
- A well-educated person who has a good knowledge in Economics.
- He knows the basic needs of his constituents such as Health, Education, Employment, Housing, etc. and knows how to manage them adequately well.
- He has a good experience in governmental work and has a proven good track record in governance.

- He should be an emotionally stable person who is calm or relax amidst crisis situation.
- A model loving family man with no vices.
- A cultured person who appreciates the arts, music, etc.
- He should be perceptive and a good decision-maker, which are important in governmental function.
- But most of all, he is a God-fearing person who truly practices his religion faithfully well.

These essential features are to be found in a good electoral candidate who promises to render a good service and performance in government work.

Note: Please be aware of any government leader who is too blindly ambitious, too ego-centric, a braggart and a delusional or superstitious candidate.

Discipline

"Self-discipline is the bedrock of
all successful pursuits in life."
Anonymous

Filipinos have varied traits-some are too unreasonably strict and rigid, some are so lax, egocentric and unruly, while others are humble, kind and well adjusted. Why is this so? Let us learn the factors that made them so.

No nation can ever become progressive and successful in its goals without the basic element of discipline among its people.

Discipline literally means **"to learn."** Discipline is the process of learning to adapt one's behavior to the requirement of society.

Naturally, the child cannot be relied on to teach himself to curb his impulses and to conform to rules and regulations. He has to be taught by others. This teaching, however, satisfies many of his own inner needs. It helps him what is expected of him, protects him from his own destructive urges and gives him a sense of security by letting him know how far he can go and what he must do to win the approval of others.

Psychologists claim that there are three major types of discipline:

1. The **Authoritarian Approach.** This kind of discipline is characterized by a demanding, strict rule and regulation, enforced by severe punishment. The end result of this type of discipline is it rises to rankling resentment and the child becomes timid, apathetic, as well as rebellious, hostile and vindictive. This is not a good discipline.

2. The **Permissive Approach.** This kind could hardly be called discipline at all since the parents make little attempt to set limits to the child's behavior or even give him the guidance he needs. This over permissiveness will lead to feelings of insecurity and resentment for there is no consistent guidance and the child feels that his parents do not care about him. So, he becomes confused what to do. He becomes egocentric, self-assertive and spoiled. This is not a good method to adapt.

3. The **Democratic Technique Approach.** This kind of discipline is from an educational point of view. Parents make use of explanation, discussion and reasoning to help the child understand why he is expected to conduct

himself in certain ways. Good behavior is generally rewarded with praise and encouragement and bad behavior is punished only when it is willfully done. The punishment, however, is never harsh, and usually takes the form of scolding or reprimanding, deprivation of privileges, or a quick slap, or whipping at the buttock with a slipper or belt but not to be accompanied with name calling like "stupid" nor a threat of total rejection. This type of discipline encourages self-discipline and a better adjusted person in the society.

Time Management

*"To effectively manage time is
to be able to control time."*
                                Anonymous

Since childhood we were taught that "time is gold" and should be used wisely. In other words, we have to be time-conscious. Time is so precious in one's undertaking in life. People who do not know how to budget their time well would suffer greatly from the deadly stresses of living. Admittedly, we, Filipinos are poor time-conscious people. Someone said that TIME is really the only capital that any human being has and the only thing that he can't afford to lose.

Experts have found 10 valuable and effective elements in time management that should be learned an deeply instilled in their habit as people.

1. MAKE A PLAN. Start the day by making a general schedule with emphasis on two or

three important things you like to accomplish. Prioritize them and set deadlines.

2. CONCENTRATE. Do not be interrupted in doing too many things at once. Do it piece-meal or think one thing at a time on the most important task.

3. TAKE A BREAK. Relieve tension by doing isometric exercise like walking around, deep breathing, stretching or going to the restroom. You may take a light merienda. (However, "taking a break" to most Filipinos is eating a heavy snack!) You have 10 minutes for this.

4. AVOID CLUTTER. A disarrayed table or room could hinder concentration, creates tension and frustration. Put and use a wastebasket near your table or corner of your room.

5. DON'T BE A PERFECTIONIST. To strive for excellence is attainable, gratifying and healthy, but not for perfection, which is often unattainable, frustrating and a waste of time.

6. DON'T BE AFRAID TO SAY "NO!" This is a time-saving attitude. Avoid counterproductive talks–– like answering unimportant calls, uncalled for requests (i.e. *paalayon* or favors), etc. Don't worry about offending others' annoying requests.

7. DON'T PROCRASTINATE. (The "manana habit.") By all means, cut this bad habit now. "Never postpone for tomorrow what you can do today" is the best policy.

8. APPLY "RADICAL SURGERY." This sounds like a surgeon removing a pre-cancerous growth. Please stop your time-wasting activities--e.g. uncalled for socializing, "tsismis" (gossiping),

reading fantastic comics, etc. All these non-essential things will consume precious time.

9. LEARN TO DELEGATE. You don't have to be the boss all the time. You must educate and trust your subordinates and assign them some tasks to facilitate routine matters. This decision will lessen your work load and saves time.

10. DON'T BE A "WORKAHOLIC." Workaholic is a guy who is addicted to his work to get rich quick. He refuses to relax and avoid taking a vacation.

There should be a time for everything. The book entitled "The Spice of Life" compiled by Dian Ritter contains several quotations about the value of time. These are the following tenets:

- Take time to THINK-it is the source of power.
- Take time to PLAY-it is the secret of perpetual youth.
- Take time to be FRIENDLY-it is the road to happiness.
- Take time to READ--it is the fountain of wisdom.
- Take time to LAUGH-it is the music of the soul.
- Take time to GIVE-it is too short a day to be selfish.
- Take time to WORK-it is the price of success.
- Take time to EXERCISE-it is the pillar of strength and health.
- Take time to LOVE-it is a God-given privilege.
- Take time to PRAY-it is the greatest power on earth.

The above 10 meaningful tenets are considered the best basic human guide and a brief summary of valuable principles that every responsible person, a true Christian must learn and internalize to practice consistently to be able to achieve fully and fulfill the ultimate personal health, happiness and success that we always strive in this life.

Undoubtedly, <u>counseling</u> can help people cope with time conflicts. Pray to God, the Alpha and the Omega of Time for guidance.

Kindness

> *"Any kindness that I can show to any*
> *human being let me do it now for*
> *I shall not pass this way again."*
> Anonymous

Kindness is one of the most precious virtues of man. This great moral fortitude has been exemplified a number of times in the Holy Scriptures, such as the Good Samaritan, who truly helped a wounded and dying stranger along his way; the father of the prodigal son, who unconditionally welcomed him home despite his grievous offense; kindness was tangibly shown when a prostitute knelt in front of Jesus and wept, her tears falling on His feet. The woman wiped the tears with her hair and kissed His feet and washed them with perfume. Although she was a great sinner, with her kindest acts, *"She loved me much."* And He said to her, *"Your sins are forgiven...your faith has saved you. Go in peace."* (Luke 7:36-50, NKJV)

Kindness is the sincere intention of doing good things towards a person or oneself. It is synonymous to benevolence, amiability, thoughtfulness, and altruism. The pure manifestation of kindness of a truly benevolent person is the fact that he does not count the cost and does not expect anything in return. All genuine philanthropies are made of such stuff. They are God-sent people. May their tribe increase.

Sages say that no act of kindness, no matter how small, is ever wasted. It is very important that parents should teach their children to be kind to others.

There are many ways one can show kindness to our fellowmen. This is well expressed in the Holy *Gospel-*
"Share your Time, Talent and Treasure to your neighbors."
We can do this by:

- Helping in many ways our indigent neighbors.
- Sparing time to plant trees in flood-prone areas in our community.
- Participating in "car pool" to let some people ride in your car to the city.
- Make a habit of "Picking up" trash you see along your way.
- Donate any amount in the drop box of the needy, etc.
- Let us always pray St. Frances of Asissi's Prayer of Benevolence: *"Lord make me an instrument of peace..."* Loving kindness is what unites us as Christians.

The True Spirit of Giving

*"It is more blessed to give
than to receive."*
Acts 20:35, KJV

In the Season of Giving, everybody is inspired to greet one and all-"Merry Christmas." Our Mother Church has designated a "Year of the Poor." Apparently, our marginalized brothers have long been neglected, exploited, and abandoned in their lives by the rich segment in our society. Hence, the poor remain in their destitute state while the rich become filthy rich.

The Holy Scripture clearly says: "He who gives to the poor will lack nothing, but he who closes his eyes to them will receive many curses." (Proverbs 28:27, NKJV) Here is the most painful consequence of selfishness, which is truly exemplified in the Holy Bible: When Lazarus, the Poor Man died he went straight to heaven in the bosom of Abraham while the Greedy Rich Man went to hell, tormented.

The existential question: What will I give when I have nothing to give? Giving is not only confined to material things. The Holt Bible emphatically says: "Share willingly your Time, Talent, Treasure." The perfect example is the Parable of the Good Samaritan. Therefore, if we are conscious of our moral and social obligations towards our family and neighbors, this world will be a much better place to live.

A beautiful reminder: "Each man should give what his heart desires to give, not reluctantly or under compulsion, for God is Cheerful Giver!" (2 Corinthians 8:9, NKJV)

Don't be a Scrooge! (From Christmas Carol by Charles Dickens.)

Handicap is not a Hindrance to Success

Here is a true dictum in life-"Where you fall, there you must stand." This is a very correct statement. If we apply this truism to those who failed in their first attempts, you will be truly inspired.

Let me mention a few who were able to conquer their weaknesses and became successful in the end.

Charles Atlas, a skinny kid who hated the way he looked. He was always bullied by bigger boys of his age. He discovered the "Dynamic Tension" and developed a perfect body and strongest strength.

Abraham Lincoln, a politician who lost in the election for seven times. He ran again and at last he won. He became one of the best American presidents.

Joan of Arc, an ordinary peasant girl who served as a soldier to a French King. Because of her good works and loyalty to the King, she was made to lead the Army for war and became successful because they won in the battle. The American Helen Keller, born deaf and blind, became a good writer and a philanthropist.

The above mentioned names are good examples of people who conquered their disabilities and utter failures to human successes, respectively.

A lot of gifted people have tried investing or developing something in life but failed or became failures in their first attempts. Most of them easily gave up and never attempted to try again. The worse thing for those who have no guts-they go into depression and the worst thing, some end up to committing suicide.

Remember: FAILURE IS A GOOD STARTING POINT.

THANKFULNESS-Gratitude at its Best

*"Give thanks in all circumstances for
this is God's will for you in Jesus Christ."*
1 Thessalonians 5:18 NIV

Essentially, all of us were created by the Almighty God with a good purpose. In this sense, we are therefore, obliged to reciprocate this divine privilege to worship and thank Him for all the days of our lives.

In the Old Testament, righteous people who received some blessings from God had always manifested their sincere gratitude by offering. As the Greek writer Seneca said: "Nothing is more honorable than a grateful heart." Also an anonymous writer said: "Ingratitude is sharper than a serpent's tooth." In the Holy Scripture, an incident happened when Jesus cured ten lepers but only one came back to thank Him. This proves that there are many thoughtless people in this world.

Gratitude is universally considered as one of the theological virtues belonging to love or charity. When a person expresses his thankfulness, thoughtfulness, or care after receiving something of value, certainly, we can say that this person is good, kind, respectful, and understanding.

The year 2011 has ended and many of our people should be thankful to Almighty God for the countless blessings that they have received in life. We have to be truly thankful to God that majority of our province mates have been spared and saved from the devastating typhoon Sendong where many lives and properties were lost and destroyed in just a day.

Thankfulness is a virtue every person who wants to succeed in life should have.

The Value of a Smile

"A smile costs nothing, but gives much."
Anonymous

One of the most beautiful songs ever composed is "Smile" sung by Nat King Cole in the late 50's. This meaningful song is often the theme song played during weddings and anniversaries to bring back and reminisce the endearing moment of a lifetime. To most sensible writers a "smile brings courage, sunshine to the sad, and a good medicine for troubled minds."

Studies have shown that the limbic system of the brain is the center believed to be responsible for our emotional expression. It also produces endorphins, the happy hormones, which induces the happy feelings and the anti-pain sensation of the body. Psychologists say that the effect of a mother's smile on her baby brings a healthy emotional response of tremendous joy and security, as well as a positive mood and physical development.

Generally, a person who readily smiles is often a loving, a peaceful, and a happy person. Some people must have seen an unusual portrait of Jesus smiling that was displayed in a corridor of a convent. Certainly, that pleasant countenance of Jesus depicts the true gladness in His heart and a most friendly person.

In the science of kinesis (body language), a smile is a facial gesture, which means "welcome, agreement, or appreciation." A real smile gladdens the heart and reaches up and crinkles the eyes. But a fake smile looks more like a grimace and usually indicates trouble or dishonesty. Only bad people have scornful and sarcastic smiles on their faces.

There are various kinds of smiles that are shown to depict happiness. For instance, the enigmatic smile, called as "mystifying smile" of Mona Lisa, as painted by Leonardo da Vinci; the triumphant smile of a champion after a close fight; the smile of a surgeon after a successful surgery of a difficult case; the bright smile of a mother after a hard labor; the splendid smile of a student after passing a difficult board examination; and so on.

A beautiful saying on smile goes-"If you meet the world with a smile, the world will always smile back at you." Christians are often reminded to carry their crosses with a smile. But most humans, generally, would rather "cry" than smile when they are carrying a heavy load on their shoulders. But there are few individuals who welcome sufferings we call "moral masochists" those who can truly endure pain and long fasting. There are saintly or martyrs in this world.

So, let us train our lips to often smile like "painting the dark cloud with sunshine." A smile always adds something of value to our "poker" face and wins the admiration of friends and foes alike. Remember that a smile is an anti-stress element that enhances beauty, health, and longer life. If you want a winning personality and succeed in life-- SMILE!

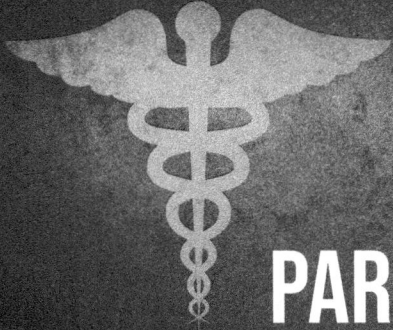

PART XI

ALL ABOUT CHILDREN'S HEALTH AND BEHAVIOR

Parental Lesson for the Child's Character Development

Sages say that education of the human mind should start from the cradle. Hence, parents are relegated by the Almighty God the prime responsibility and sacred duty in molding the character of their children. And definitely every growing child needs proper guidance. Therefore, parents should be fully aware of the essential factors direly needed in the formation of child's character.

Authorities aptly define character as the ultimate development of a good conscience, moral concepts, social attitudes, and religious values. As a consequence, consistent parenting should be able to make the child discern between what is "right and wrong." Hopefully, the child would become a righteous and law-abiding citizen in the future.

The most indispensable factors needed of character formation as studies have shown are:

1. Parents should be able to live a simple kind of life, coupled with a peaceful and loving relationship with their children. They should realize that true happiness in life is "not in getting more but in wanting less." A too material life is evil.

2. A righteous parent should truly possess the Christian values of love, joy, discipline, peace, honesty, diligence, responsibility, kindness, humility, forgiveness, fervent spirituality (Christ-centered life).

3. Never let your child see you quarrel frequently. This will give him a bad example for his own future marriage.

4. Be sure to make you rules in the family very clear to be fully understood by every child. Be firm and learn to say "No" to an impulsive and insistent child whose desire may lead to a disastrous ending.

5. Know how to appreciate or praise and duly reward every child who meritoriously shows his/her true creative talent or any commendable behavior. This will positively bolster his self-esteem and justifiable pride.

6. Parents are duty-bound to reasonably admonish (counsel) and fairly punish a truly erring child. This corrective and disciplinary act must be tempered with love. As the wise saying goes, "Bend the tree while still young." Expect an upright adult in the future.

7. Avoid nagging, fault-finding and criticizing the child for his honest mistake nor scolding him in front of his friends and or people. This

definitely will destroy his precious self-esteem and he will become angry and rebellious.

8. Never bribe the child for any favor duly done, but just express your sincere thanks and he will be happy, indeed.
9. Stop the bad parental habit of overprotecting the child known as "over palangga system." This perennial practice will foster a negative feeling of inadequacy and inferiority complex in the child.
10. Conscientious parents must instill and nurture an ardent sense of spirituality in the heart and soul of every child under their consistent and loving care.

Be happy, good and responsible parents because the crowning glory, which is Heaven awaits you for a job well done!

Parent-Child Relationship

"We never know the love of the parents till we become parents ourselves."
Quote by Henry Ward Beecher

One of the greatest lessons of love I learned from a close friend and pastor from a well-known university is: "Next to God, the parents."

I am a believer of what Pope John Paul II said-"In God's plan there is no such thing as chance." God is absolutely omniscient. Definitely, He knows everything even before we were born. Some philosophers even dared say: "How may zygotes (fertilized eggs) have been flashed down the toilet bowls because God knows that if He'll let them live and grow, these persons to be will become "evil genius" and certainly be damned to hell. We are more privileged to be born, to know, to love, and to serve God through our parents.

Parental experts claim that to be a good and consistent parent is a difficult task. There is no such thing as perfect parent. There are vital factors that guide a parent towards good and consistent parenting. These essential elements include: love, discipline, fairness, honesty, avoidance of negative criticism, right praising, reward and punishment, etc. However, it is difficult to maintain consistency in all these measures. But a very important and lasting factor that every Christian parent could bequeath to his children is the true development of their spirituality-God-fearing and God-centered life. Mature parents should be conscious that all mortals will die sooner or later and their souls will be finally judged fairly. One certain question God will ask: "Did you love your parents as I love you? Or hate and condemn them for their past mistakes?"

The parable of "The Prodigal Son" is truly a convincing Lesson of Love of a father towards a wayward son. In the same manner, we should love our parents and never condemn them of whatever "crime or mistakes" they have committed. Develop a true forgiving heart-a mark of an Authentic Christian!

Separation Anxiety

Separation anxiety is defined as the infant's vague and persistent apprehension of the loss of its mother. This feeling of dread and loss of one's mother is generally felt by the child when he enters preschool and left in the classroom to join with other kids and to be taken care of by the teacher who is now the "surrogate mother." Majority of the children when enrolled in the preschool have no problem. They can join with other kids and adjust easily with the classmates and teacher in the class. However, there are also some children who *are* seriously suffering from separation anxiety. They cannot be left alone in the classroom with other kids. Hence, the mother or "yaya" has to stay with the anxious child in the class until the class is over. This ordeal will last several days, weeks, or even months.

There are also adults who *are* suffering from "separation anxiety." They *are* so attached with their mother. Hence, they can never get out of their mother's life. They *are* perpetually known as children with an unresolved separation anxiety. They *are* extremely disturbed, tense, sleepless and anxious.

Child psychiatrists have found a procedure of resolving the problem of separation anxiety of a child. This is the playful method of "Pick-a-boo." You say: "Close your eyes. You don't see me." And then: "Open your eyes. Now, I'm here again." Repeat the same procedure until the child will realize and can master separation anxiety.

In adulthood, we lessen the "pang" of long separation through simple process of celebrating a party together, taking pictures, exchanging gifts, and other rituals...like sending off for departing relatives and friends.

In life, we always master reunion and separation–– there is the hello...and the goodbye!!!

God bless us.

Why Children Rebel

Children are the best gift parents receive from God. Parents are given the task of molding their children's total development from their health of body, mental attitude, emotional and spiritual well-being. The bottom line of all this formation is consistent discipline coupled with loving care. Parents should always spend quality time with their children, not matter how busy they are. Parents should make their rules clear and must apply them well. They should know how to punish and reward their children properly.

I know of a friend, a successful businessman whose children were subjected to a "strict discipline" when they were growing up. All of them graduated Cum laude in their college course, respectively at UST, Manila. They are a happy family. They always go to church together.

It cannot be denied that there are also families whose children don't have good relationship with their parents so much so that they become delinquent in their homes and later in the society. Why is this so?

Here are a number of factors that could be traced back as to why children rebel against their parents:

- Absence of parental care because parents are working abroad.
- Most of the children are under the care of people who are also working for a living, and these care-takers are not strict in disciplining the children. They cannot control them.
- When these children, whose allowance are big, would go out to enjoy with their barkadas, they would just spend the whole night or day in places where they enjoy pot sessions.
- Most of these children who were already dependent with marijuana will now graduate to take "Shabu" peddled around.
- All of these children are enjoying the **Online**

Games, playing the whole night in stations they like to promenade.

- If they are enrolled in a school, they become truants. Hence, most of them are "drop-outs."
- When the parents come home these children show their outward resentment and hostility towards them. Some do not come home anymore.
- If parents could not send enough money, they would sell a lot of things from their homes, or pawn them. Many are involved in gun-running and smuggling things.
- Many would become antisocial personality and worse, would become victims of extrajudicial killings!

Sibling Rivalry

> *"Sibling rivalry is a kind of silent war (crisis) that exists between children in the family."*
>
> Anonymous

Generally, parents are worried when their own children show some hostile feelings against each other and certainly, they are at a loss as to how to handle the serious conflict at hand. Some of these problems may escalate to a very serious proportion that the antagonistic feeling of hostility and vindictiveness will be carried until adulthood or even to the end of their lives.

Psychologists say that sibling rivalry is a normal and inevitable occurrence that happens in every family of two or more children. The situation may be observed during early childhood. In young children, it may take the direct and open form. For example, upon the birth of another baby, the elder sibling may act queerly like crying very loudly, refuses to eat, or show some tantrums. Some worse manifestations, an extreme reaction of an insecure child is defecating anywhere. This unpleasant behavior is directed towards the hated mother and an indirect call for attention to Care for him and not to his newborn brother or sister. The elder child has a fantasy that he will be "dethroned" (usurp) as the first favorite child. Later on the older insecure child may tease, hit, punch or mock at the younger brother or sister and the younger child may complain against the older brother. Older siblings may always quarrel on pity matters.

Clearly, sibling rivalry usually originates in competition for the mother's affection and attention. This occurs commonly at the age of two or so. These feelings are likely to be particularly acute in children who are possessive and demanding tendencies which sometimes stem from parental favoritism or indulgence such as the *palangga* (the favored one) system of the Filipinos.

Parents should understand that children are good observers. Children often mistakenly believe that only one person in a family can have a certain claim to fame. For instance, the eldest child usually tries to be first and the boss; the second child looks for the injustices and tries hard to catch up with the first; the youngest child thinks he is entitled to extra attention; and the only child wants to be special all the time. The kids will find their own ways to belong and feel significant. Parents should tell each child that it is okay to feel jealous.

How then can sibling rivalry be reduced?

- By making each child feel to be fully loved and accepted unconditionally.
- By encouraging them to develop their own

interests, activities and friends. Stress group cooperation and teamwork in work and play.
- Do not compare the kids or pick favorites.
- Gradually help children realize that each one has special abilities, rights and prerogatives that set them apart from other kids.

Make sure that the message of LOVE gets through with each child for being a unique human being that he or she is.

The Significance of Loving Touch

"We all need a hug."

Anonymous

The famous American psychologist, Abraham Maslow, has categorized human needs. The most important physical and physiological needs are things that make us alive-food, shelter, clothing, motion (exercise), sex, etc. But Maslow's third hierarchy of human need is what he calls as the need for **love, touch, self-esteem, and acceptance.**

We all need to be loved. Definitely, an affectionate relationship without love will make us all feel empty and lonely human beings. If the child is not loved and cuddled or cared consistently by the mother, that child will suffer from severe mental and emotional disorders.

Studies have consistently shown that every infant who is always cuddled, tenderly touch by the mother will result to healthy growth and development physically and mentally.

Modern parents practice and allow their children to kiss the older relatives, male or female on the lips instead of kissing the hand, a more hygienic way. Fathers should decide not to nestle on their lap their daughter to prevent malicious erotic movement. Mothers should stop bathing their older boys or cleaning their private parts. Young widowed mothers should not sleep together in the same bed to prevent erotization or stimulation.

As your boy or girl reaches adolescence, his or her dormant sexual drive is easily aroused. Hence, dating must be controlled and properly done. Adolescence are knowledgeable on sexual matters through the Internet and other Mass Media. Hence, pregnancy among adolescence is increasing. Most students are now exposed to close physical relationship and engaging in too much kissing, which escalate to necking and petting.

Let us hold hands together and pray to God for our dear life!

What is Pedophilia?

In any known society there are individuals who prefer to sexually molest children instead of adults. We often observe and read in the newspapers reported cases of children being sexually abused by hedonistic foreign nationals and by Filipino male sex offenders. They usually victimized children who are easily attracted or lured by their generosity and attention to their needs in all aspects in order to gain the victims' trust, affection, interest and loyalty. The child offender or pedophile usually does this manipulation to prevent the innocent child from reporting the abnormal sexual activity to any authority.

Pedophilia literally means love of children. Its psychiatric definition of the term is the <u>recurrent,</u>

<u>intense, sexual urges and sexually arousing fantasies or behaviors involving sexual activity with a child who has not reached puberty (before adolescence)</u>. The pedophile has acted on these urges or is markedly distressed by them. Studies of pedophilia show that those attracted to girls usually prefer 8 to 10 years old, where as those attracted to boys usually prefer slightly older children. Attraction to girls is apparently twice as common as attraction to boys. Many pedophiliac are sexually aroused by both young boys and young girls.

Pedophiles who act on their urges with children may limit their activity to undressing the child and looking, exposing themselves, masturbating in the presence of the child or gently touching and fondling the child. Others performed fellatio (licking or sucking the male organ) or cunnilingus (licking or sucking of the female organ) of the child or attempt intercourse or penetrate the child's vagina, mouth or anus with their fingers, foreign objects or penis and use varying degrees of force to achieve these ends. These activities are commonly explained with excuses or rationalizations that they have educational value for the child, that the child derives sexual pleasure from them or that the child is sexually provocative--themes that are common in pedophilic pornography.

It is believed that many pedophiles were themselves victims of sexual abuse in their childhood.

Today, reliable reports of children in big cities like Manila, Cebu, etc. are victims of cybersex crimes for commercial purposes.

Pedophilia is a very serious offense. And the perpetrators should be put to prison!

The High Risks of the Online World

"He that loveth pleasure
shall be a poor man."
Proverbs 21:17, KJV

There was a time before when innocent people were delighted and thought that when their children play harmless games on the internet, they thought that things were alright. But the big question arises, "Why are our children not doing well in school?"

Today, reports are alarming and parents must be aware of the evil consequences of the addictive online gaming. Of course, many garners think that these games are teaching themselves skills. But here's the irony-online gaming never sleeps. Even at midnight up to the wee hours of dawn, youngsters would still not sleep because they are so much obsessed with it and its fantasy world. They need to get a life, a sense of reality.

The Internet, a multimedia provider, also has its cons. Most minors, especially boys, are exposed to adult content through movies, pictures and video streams provided by the Internet. Definitely, these vicarious things will seriously affect their way of thinking, resorting to violence. Their performance in school will drastically deteriorate, failing in class and refuse to function properly. What's worse is that many have been victimized by sinister and cunning strangers through social networks, targeting women, especially teenagers for sex. First they'll introduce themselves as "friends" but once a youngster is totally convinced by the "smooth and sweet talker," then she is enticed and captured within his clutches, leaving her vulnerable.

This "Romeo" will start inviting the gullible girl and once she goes out alone and is mesmerized by the stranger, it's game over. Kidnapping her in the process and dragging her away for prostitution. If she tries to resist, she could be murdered.

Well, this is only one of the tragic episodes that happen here and abroad. Certainly, we are living in a Cyberspace Age and Satan, taking it to his advantage and even using it as a convenient tool for moral destruction of our naive and innocent youth. Of course, most of our smart children would readily rationalize-"Okay lang. I'm old enough to do things!" But don't be fooled, smart kid, the devil is smarter than you! Remember, regrets come last.

Suggestion: Parents must teach, control and discipline their children on HOW LONG and HOW THEY SPEND THEIR TIME ONLINE.

Mobile Phone Affects Brain Function

A Health News Medical update recently reports an alarming warning finding which claims that mobile phone affects the brain of the user.

Scientists study from Swinburne University of Technology's and Brain Science Institute in Melbourne, Australia found that user's reaction response time slowed down during a 30-minute mobile phone call.

The researchers conducted a series of psychological test on 120 volunteers as they were exposed to mobile phone emissions for half an hour. The neuropsychologists showed a discernable change in brain function among those who were exposed to the electromagnetic fields that phone mobiles generate.

People who use the mobile phone a lot seem to have more of impairment than people who are not frequent users.

Well, we are aware of the adverse effects of too much radiation effects of X-ray exposure. Hence, in the same manner, we have to minimize the exposure of mobile phones electromagnetic field. **Remember:** An ounce of prevention is better than a pound of cure.

The lesson is: **Don't ever abuse your cell phone.** Use it only sparingly when needed, OK? Always protect your brain, man!

The Evil Effects of Television Violence on Our Children

"Nothing good ever comes from violence."
Martin Luther

Incidentally, some American Psychologists suggest that violence in cartoons can help children mold their character positively. But a sensitive parent should always think that any violence should always be rejected.

Today, mass media through television shows, online games through the Internet, and cinema greatly contribute to the formation of the character of our innocent children. Of course, the main aim of T.V. or movie producers is to educate the audience, one way or another, for an enormous economic interest and gain. Children readily absorb what they hear and see, favorable or unfavorable to their senses. They tend to imbibe not only the positive side of the role models but also the negative aspects that are depicted to add to the realism of the show.

Most children are attracted to the thrills of excessive and bloody combats like the gory killings of one's enemy, the escaping away from prison, the stealing of precious jewels and other smart moves that defy the law or authorities like "Catch me if you can." Most cartoons show unrealistic scenes enhancing or exaggerating fantasy and mystery like magical phenomena, which truly mesmerize the child's imagination transporting the child to a make-believe world like a dreamland. Hence, many children love to see "Harry Potter" movies for the adventure, magic and witches.

Bust most T.V. shows and movies today glorify sex and violence. Undoubtedly, cybercrimes and many of the crimes like killings (shootings), stealing, smuggling, drug abuse, alcoholism, rape, sexual immorality, corruption (cheatings), human trafficking of our youth are strongly shown. These crimes are definitely influencing their psyche consciously or unconsciously.

How to Keep Our Children Safe from Harm

Children by nature are basically curious, restless and impulsive. They are potentially vulnerable to harm and accidents. Besides, they are so unpredictable. Hence, parents need to control and guide them all the time.

Authorities suggest sound ways to keep our children from harm:

1. It is important to provide your growing children with a good, healthy and responsible "yaya" (nanny).
2. Be sure to keep all medicines locked in a medicine cabinet or out of reach of children.
3. Tell your children that even if medicines taste sweet, they are not "candies" (Explain).
4. Never transfer harmful or poisonous chemicals or substances into soda bottles or jars. They might be mistaken for soft drinks or edibles.

5. Put away all dangerous liquids like bleaches, polishers, acids, etc. out of reach of children.
6. Don't let your children play in isolated places where bad elements like pedophiles or kidnappers prowl.
7. Don't let your children play in or near construction sites. They can be injured or killed by falling objects.
8. Don't let your children swim alone in pools without the watchful eyes of a lifesaver. Let them use a life vest.
9. Do not force your child to ride on that high-risk roller coaster. They are too risky and scary.
10. Don't let your teenage girl join any party without a responsible chaperon. Be strict on curfews!
11. The too liberal-minded parents who give too much freedom to their "smart" adolescent are shocked to find out that their child is involved in drug abuse, alcoholism and other immoral or illegal activities. Hence, it pays to be reasonably strict but loving disciplinarian.

Remember: "A family that prays together stays together." (Fr. Patrick Payton.)

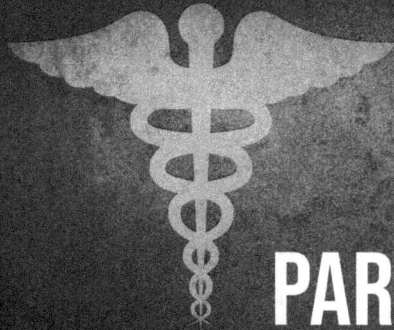

PART XII

SPIRITUALITY IN THE HEALING PROCESS

The Healing Power of Faith

> *"Faith is to believe what we do not see, and the reward of this faith is to see what we believe."*
>
> St. Augustine

As we journey through the crossroads of life, we still find ourselves in a great quandary, despite our knowledge and rationality. We are still confronted with existential questions of which there are no ready answers. Man must need a strong and unwavering faith to understand the various paradoxes of life. Otherwise, he gets lost in the labyrinth of complexities of this world. The Swiss psychologist, Carl G. Lung said, "Without faith, life has not meaning." As a Christian doctor, I never doubted for a moment, the awesome power of faith in the healing process. There is a saying which goes, "The doctor treats the illness but God heals." True, Jesus heals and makes our bodies temple of the Holy Spirit.

Let us first define what faith is. Generally, faith means one's religious belief, creed, sect or church. Ordinarily, we refer faith as trust, confidence, reliance, or assistance. It could also mean a verbal pledge, premise, word of honor or loyalty. In this particular issue, I would like to focus on the amazing healing power of faith.

It is a common observation and experience in life that every human being is vulnerable to the devastating "life events" that often trigger anxiety, depression and the feeling of hopelessness following a serious heart attack, cancerous growth, crippling accidents and its complications. However, people with deep faith have the steadfast tenacity that somehow Almighty God, the Divine Healer, eventually help them cope with the overwhelming crisis that have adversely affected them. Undoubtedly, this is the answer to their fervent prayers and as if a "miracle" has happened, physical healing takes place. What an amazing grace, indeed! Scientific studies of faith's healing potential have come out with convincing evidence that strong religious faith not only promotes overall good health but also aids in recovering from serious illnesses.

An American researcher, Dr. Koenig, observed that religious patients, when praying to God, acquired an indirect form of control over their illnesses. He also found in his studies that people who attend church services, like Holy Mass, healing ministries, etc., spent fewer days in a hospital than people who rarely attend church services. Researchers in the U.S. and other countries found that after a heart surgery, people who were not religious died within six months, but unbelievably, no death among people who professed they were deeply religious. Another study revealed that elderlies who never attend church had nearly twice the stroke rate than the weekly churchgoers.

Many studies of healing through strong faith have

remarkably shown that relaxed state brought on by prayers and meditations reduces the impact of stress hormones and adrenaline. Repetitive prayers lower the blood pressure and even slow the brain waves, all without drugs.

Prayers will enhance the emotional comfort of the faithful. Hence, most Christian doctors realize the value of religion in the healing process. We are just instruments in the "ultimate healing experience."

Remember that human life is God's miracle and He made our bodies Temple of the Holy Spirit.

The Awesome Power of Prayer

"When good people pray,
the Lord listens."
Proverbs 15:29, GNT

Theologians all over the world assert that prayer is the most important aspect of any religion. Through the ages, it has taken various forms as an expression of worshipping, praising and thanking God.

What is prayer? Prayer is simply defined as an earnest request or a plea to God. It is synonymous with supplication or entreaty. Prayer is our direct communication with our Savior. Great men have their beautiful concept of prayer. "Prayer is the voice of faith." (Heme); "Prayer is not asking. It is the language of the soul." (Gandhi); "Prayer is my journey towards God." (Fr. Leo Booth).

Why do we pray? Reasonably, we are all created by God with a good purpose. God has saved us from the eternal damnation in hell by dying ignominiously on the cross. We owe God our very life. All martyrs and saints have lived in a prayerful lives. Jesus is the most prayerful person.

Responsible parents have emphasized the importance of prayer to their children and taught them how to pray. It was the late American, Rev. Fr. Patrick Peyton, who propagated the well-known "Family Rosary Crusade" with its slogan: "The family that prays together, stays together." This motto definitely strengthened the bond of family solidarity throughout the world.

Personally, I have always prayed to my Guardian Angel. Undoubtedly, he saved me from a number of horrifying near-death experiences in my life. Dr. Albert Shiebert in his book "Survivor Personality," attested that all survivors (believers and non-believers) who underwent near-death episodes truly claimed that prayer definitely helped them survived. "God certainly had a hand in making us alive."

The Lord's Prayer is the best known Christian prayer of all times, It contains the sum-total of religious principles for righteous living. Prayer is a precious gift from God.

When do we pray? When we pray, we tell God our troubles and feelings. When we find work, we say a prayer of thanksgiving; when we get sick, we say a prayer of healing; when in trouble, ask God for help; when sad due to heavy burden, ask God to lighten the load; when faced with a problem, pray for wisdom and understanding; when we have sinned, pray for forgiveness; when weary and weak, pray for strength. We have to pray for others, for our basic needs, for peace, etc.

There are essential things to remember when we pray. First, we need to have a close and deep relationship with God. Second, we must sincerely and humbly open up to God from our heart. Thirdly, we have to be specific in our prayer and request. Finally, firmly believe that our prayer will be answered. "Thy will be done Oh Lord."

Pray fervently and unceasingly to reassure our sanctity.

The Healing Power of Doing Good

The healing power of doing good or altruism as the Holy Bible emphasizes like sharing one's time, talent and treasure are assured in the scriptural passage: "Charity covers a multitude of sins."

Altruism is an attitude of being benevolent, considerate, unselfish or kind extended to another person. The best example of an altruistic behavior was exemplified by Jesus Christ during His public life; like healing the sick, forgiving the sinners, saving people from embarrassment in His first Miracle at the Wedding at Cana. He mingled with the sinners, and at the end, He converted them. Another altruistic behavior was also exemplified by Mother Teresa of Calcutta and her congregation by helping the dire needs of the destitute and the dying.

And now in Dumaguete City, a man by the name of Estaneslao Alviola, a Negrense who is getting so popular doing an altruistic activity, giving nebulizers, medicines and vitamins to the different barangays in the City with a simple reason: out of gratitude he wants to share the blessings he has received from the Almighty to the people around him, without expecting any return or reward, that in so doing these people who are the recipients of the blessing shared will also give Glory to the Almighty. He is doing this not for political reason, as what others might think.

To God be the Glory!

The Value of Meditation

*"Creating a state of mindfulness
is a prelude to meditation and
contemplative prayer."*
Dr. Paul Meirer (Christian Psychiatrist)

Psychiatrists say that mindfulness is a meditative state that we use and practice at all times in our life. It is about fixing or focusing our attention in the present where God is. People usually associate meditation to highly spiritually endowed persons like the mystics or contemplatives.

History tells us that meditation was used by mystics centuries ago, but it was gradually forgotten by people when modern medicine came in and people became too materialistic and preoccupied in their daily living.

Today, we are entering into a new reawakening and revival in the scientific understanding of the mechanism in which faith; strong belief and positive imagination can actually unlock the mysteries and secrets of healing.

Many stress and healing centers in the world today have learned meditation not from the church but from the Eastern religious groups where avid followers take courses in transcendental meditation and relaxation techniques. For instance, breathing deeply (diaphragmatic breathing) is basically taught as a good way to begin meditation and a good sitting position is also helpful in establishing the blood flow throughout the body.

Religious authorities claim that meditation is another kind of prayer. It is a special way of using our mind they call it as **centering or focusing.** It is a very effective way of using our mind to any desirable topic, like our prayers to God to heal us from our sinfulness, from our serious illnesses, and our difficult problems in life.

A **Meditative Prayer** is the most effective way of touching the Heart of God! Sincere meditation is the way to sainthood!

Forgiveness

> *"To err is human, to forgive divine."*
> An old Adage

Faithful Christians always cite the perfect prayer of Jesus, **The Our Father.** This prayer clearly emphasizes the great significance for forgiveness-"Forgive us our trespasses as we forgive those who trespass against us." This particular prayer shows our human nature that is weak and subject to temptation incline to commit sin. This human predisposition is further confirmed by Jesus when on the cross, he cries: "Father forgive them for they do not know what they do."

We have to fully realize the immeasurable love of Almighty God when he redeemed us by His dying on the cross. He instituted the Sacrament of Penance with the sole purpose of giving a chance for sinners to repent and confess for their sins. Jesus explicitly relegated to the priests the power to forgive: "Whose sins you forgive, they are forgiven, but whose sins you retain, they are retained."

There are several episodes in the Bible when Jesus cured the physically handicapped like the blind, the lamed, the deaf, mute, the lepers, the sinners and after curing them, He would say, **"Go and sin no more."** What a feeling of tremendous relief after being healed and forgiven.

One of the greatest stories of forgiveness was the **Prodigal Son.** The father had totally forgiven his wayward son and welcomed him back to the family. Mary Magdalene was forgiven by Jesus of her grievous sins because of her great love for God.

The late Pope John Paul II was shot by a Muslim fanatic but survived the assassination attempt. When he became well, he visited the culprit in prison and pardoned him.

Mahatma Gandhi remarked, "The weak never forgive. Forgiveness is the attribute of the strong."

As Christians we have to fully realize that without forgiveness, life would be governed by an endless series of resentment, hate and retaliation.

Lord, help us hold on to the spiritual power of forgiveness. Amen.

Gaining Strength from Adversity

*"Blessed is the man who endures life's
trials for when he has stood the test,
he will be crowned with life which God
has promised to those who love Him."*
James 1:12RSV

Many have read the story of Job in the Holy Bible concerning his extreme sufferings and patience. But God rewarded him in the end. We also have learned about some individuals in life who pathetically suffered serious debilitating illness in life and later become totally paralyzed. However, despite their invalidism and practically spending most of their time in bed, they never lose hope but patiently read the Holy Scripture and books about saints and martyrs as well as other religious themes. These adversity affected individuals have fully realized the precious value of their sufferings as well as its divine reward. "Carry Your Cross with a smile." This is a courageous step that would bring them nearer to God, nearer to Heaven and Eternal life.

The psychologist Abraham Maslow describes the fact that stress will either break them down if they are weak to withstand distress, or else, they will become strong enough to endure the stress in this life.

Studies have shown that people who strive during severe disruptive changes in life commonly follow a similar pattern of actions and reactions according to Dr. Al Shievert, the author of "Survivor Personality." He claims that the victims regain emotional balance; cope during the transition, adapt in the new reality; recover to a stable condition, and thrive by learning to be better and stronger than before. But some victims feel ruined for life. Many suffer from "Post-Traumatic Stress Disorder." And their lives are never the same again. But, if the victim undergoes a consistent and long-term Psychotherapy, many of them will fully recover and strongly show self-confidence and live a better way and remain flexible and can easily cope up with any unexpected development in life.

A sensible helpful advice is, "One must know how to roll with the punches." Of course, without a strong and unwavering **faith** and a fervent **prayer,** one can never gain strength in any misfortune or crisis that may befall in life.

Best Lessons from Christian Living

> *"A useless life is an early death."*
>
> Goethe

In our transitory sojourn in this world, I would like to

share with you a few highly esteemed values that are worth achieving in this life before we finally return to dust.

1. Live the present moment. Living the present moment frees our mind from guilt, anxiety and regrets. The past is past and we don't know the future. God knows what to do with every moment of our lives.

2. It does not pay to worry. Worry does not accomplish anything except to lose our appetite, sleep and zest for living. It does not solve any problem and it only destroys our peace of mind. If we just have enough patience coupled with our ardent prayers, things get resolved.

3. We have to endure our forsakenness. Accept that life is not what we want it to be. Life is a mixture of good as well as bad times. It is a test and it is a tough one. But for those who know how to ride and adjust, survive.

4. Be first to love. This is very difficult to do for those who are offended. But Christ explicitly said, "Love your enemy." In reality, if we truly forgive and love our enemy, we will be greatly relieved from the burden of guilt and anger, which lead to our miserable distress. People who are loving and forgiving are peaceful and genuinely happy.

5. Learn to relax and have fun. After God created the world, He rested on the 7th day. When we take time to relax for even 15 minutes from work each day, we become more productive and we're easy to get along with.

6. It pays to be knowledgeable. Find time to

read inspirational books that are beneficial to your spiritual, physical and mental health such as the Holy Bible and other soul up-lifting literatures.

7. Take responsibility for your happiness. It is said that happiness is our own making. Here is a sound saying: "In order to multiply happiness, one should divide it with others."

8. Adopt a prudent philosophy in life. Philosophy that will give you meaning and direction such valuable convictions as: respecting the rights of others; helping people in time of need, and leading a well-balanced lifestyle.

9. Count your blessings and be thankful. We should always thank the Lord for all the blessings we received and protecting us from evil. The only thing God wants from us is gratefulness.

10. Always feel God's presence amidst us.....As faithful God's children, let us never forget for a moment that "when two or more are gathered together in Jesus' name, there I am in the midst." God's help is only a prayer away.

The Compatibility of Psychology and Religion

There are no contradictions between the principles of sound religion and those of sound psychology. There are at times only apparent ones, the result of some misunderstanding. Sound religion and sound psychology support and enhance each other. We should not separate them, but integrate them; not perceive them as naturally exclusive, but as complementary.

Psychology is the science that deals with the study

of the mental and behavioral development of man. <u>Religion</u> is the belief and practice of people for the welfare of their moral and spiritual needs especially for the salvation of their immortal soul (Christian view).

As a science, psychology helps us understand ourselves; religion enlightens our concept of God. Psychology explains the interactions at work in human relationship; religion emphasizes our relationship with God and with one another. Through psychology we get in touch with God.

Love God and your neighbor is the center of Christ's teaching. If I don't love myself, how can I love others and God? Psychology teaches us about loving, about pitfalls in loving, about real and imagined love. About the demands of love. Believing, accepting and trusting God requires believing, accepting and trusting ourselves. With the help of psychology we can root out the contradictions, superficiality and neurotic dimensions of our personal faith.

Psychology teaches healthy behavior, emotional wholeness and maturing growth, and how we can rise above and beyond ourselves. Christianity teaches us about redemption, reconciliation and resurrection.

Psychology can serve to foster a deeper understanding of ourselves, which will enable us to better follow Jesus.

"Think well." "Feel well." "Do well." (Pope Francis)

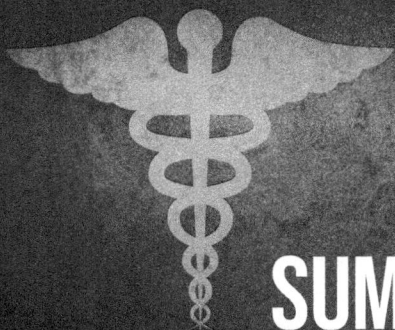

Right Mental Attitudes For Healthy Living

1. Be a POSITIVE THINKER and a truly LOVING PERSON to reassure your happiness and peace with the world. The state of mind is foremost.

2. Be sure of eating a WELL-BALANCED DIET and AVOID JUNK FOODS, TOO FATTY AND SALTY FOODS in order to guarantee a sound health and longer life.

3. Discipline yourself by AVOIDING all forms of HARMFUL VICES AND BAD HABITS that will certainly impoverish you and make you a very dependent and sickly person.

4. To be well and secured always follow the altruistic dictum of DOING THINGS IN MODERATION in everything that you do in life in order to have a satisfying result of your activity.

5. It is always beneficial for you to engage in a REGULATED FORM OF EXERCISE every day to acquire the needed strength, endurance and sturdy health against all types of diseases.

6. It is always advantageous to shield yourself

against ALL KINDS OF POLLUTIONS coming from noise, air, food, sex and water–– all stressors that eventually will cause diseases and disorders.

7. Learn to APPRECIATE WORK for it is the source of great satisfaction and self-worth. Honest work is said to be the true hallmark of success in one's life. Dislike for work and laziness will often lead to an "emotionally-induced illness."

8. Often, try to put a DASH OF HUMOR into your conversation to spice up things, because laughter is considered to be a very good tonic for boredom and sadness.

9. Endeavor to be truly MATURE PERSON--one who possesses self-discipline, self-confidence, flexibility, courage and integrity. Dr. Abraham Maslow, the American psychologist, calls this individual as a "Self-Actualizer."

10. Strive always to seek for the RIGHT COMPANIONS AND FRIENDS in your life to assure you of good influence. Avoid unreliable characters that create troubles now and then that make you regret for the rest of your life.

11. Adequate SLEEP, REST AND RELAXATION are known to be good regimen for one's health. Avoid too strenuous tasks that make you suffer overfatigue and "workaholism," for these surely predispose you to "stress-related illnesses."

12. Set aside a time for WHOLESOME RECREATION for this is very much essential for your prime health and happiness. Therefore, enjoy a meaningful hobby like listening to nice music, seeing a beautiful TV program, singing, ballroom dancing, gardening, etc.

13. Once in a while, foster a pleasant SOCIAL RELATIONSHIP with your friends and neighbors. Do not be an isolationist. Join social functions and enjoy the interactions with people. Remember, "No man is an island."

14. Be a CULTURED AND CREATIVE PERSON. Develop your aesthetic sense and God-given talents. Learn to appreciate the arts as well as the beauty of nature around you. Be an "artist" of whatever you are to inspire others.

15. Here is a good outlet for your unpleasant emotions. VERBALIZE YOUR INNER FEELINGS to a level-headed person whom you trust. Too much repression makes you vulnerable to suffer from serious mental and emotional disorders.

16. When you feel that things are getting out of bounds and you cannot cope up any longer, then make a wise decision to SEEK FOR PROFESSIONAL HELP before things become insurmountable.

17. Resolve to live EACH PASSING DAY as the "BEST AND THE LAST DAY OF YOUR LIFE." This is an excellent reminder for every living mortal who is realistically forewarned of his inescapable destiny that "death comes like a thief in the night."

18. To properly know the real state of your health, be sure to undergo a general MEDICAL CHECK-UP by a competent doctor. The aim is for preventive as well as curative purposes.

19. Adopt a SOUND PHILOSOPHY IN LIFE that will give meaning and direction in everything that you do, such as rendering genuine service to

others; sharing with the poor; respecting the rights of others; teaching the unenlightened; living a well-balanced lifestyle.

20. A very precious thing that really counts most in this life is to be a TRULY SPIRITUAL PERSON. This valuable state of being will reassure one in the quest for the salvation of his immortal soul when he finally departs from this world.

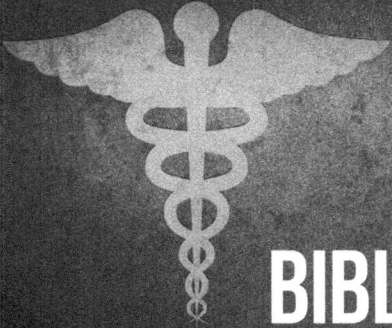

BIBLIOGRAPHY

Rod Plotnik-Introduction to Psychology, 4th Edition
Marvin R. Levy, et. al.-Life and Health, 5th Edition
Dr. Sharon S. Brehm-Social Psychology
Dr. Steven Brunton, et. al.-Encyclopedia of Medical Care
Dr. Mortimer J. Adler-Great Ideas, Great Books
Dr. Robert M. Goldenson-The Encyclopedia of Human
    Behavior
American Psychiatric Association-Psychiatry, DSM-IV
Arthur J. Snider-Nervous Tension
Dr. Ira J. Chanoff.-Family Medical Guide
Julio F. Silverio-Book of Tips
C.S. Canonigo-Sparks of Wisdom, Poems for Young
    and Adults
Catholic Bishop Conference of the Philippines-
    Catechism/or Filipino Catholics
M. Basil Pennington-Pocket Book of Prayers
Cyrus Saremi-Easy Diet
Cory Quirino-ABC of Wellness
Bernie Ward-Think Yourself Well
L.A. Justice-Healthy Moves
Ronald M. Klatz-Fight Aging
Bea Valoroso-Selected Posters
Jeffrey Laign-Slow Down Aging

Chiara Lubich-Christian Living Today
Mama Owen–– Health II ED
Modesta G. Boquiren-Quality Quotations
Diana Reyes-Stay Young and Healthy
Reader's Digest
Health Magazines (monthly Editions)
Living Words from the Holy Bible
Dr. Angel V. Somera-45 Ways of Busting Stress, "Health is Wealth" Weekly Column, Negros Chronicle

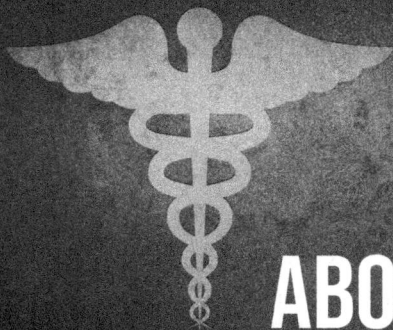

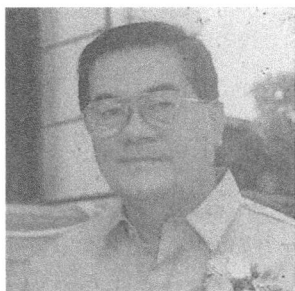

DR. ANGEL V. SOMERA, M.D., F.P.P.A., graduated from the University of Santo Tomas, College of Medicine, Manila in 1961. He specialized in Psychiatry at the University of the Philippines (UP-PGH) Medical Center in Manila. He was a former Associate Professor in Psychiatry in four Medical Schools in Cebu City, Philippines and Chief of the Provincial Psychiatric Hospital in Dumaguete City, in the province of Negros Oriental, Philippines.

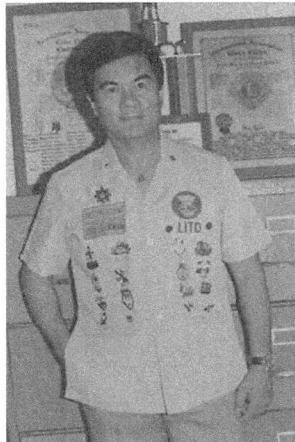

He was a Diplomate of the Philippine Board of Psychiatry and a Fellow of the Philippine Psychiatric Association. He was also a Dangerous Drugs Board Accredited Physician of the Philippines. He had attended Psychiatric Congresses and Conventions around the world and was a recipient of a "Humanitarian Service Award," plus several Special and Appreciation

Certificate Awards from various professional groups and civic organizations.

Dr. Somera has been an active socio-economic leader in his community. He was once the President of the Queen City Lions' Club of Cebu. He used to be a National Lecturer on Stress Management during Psychiatric conventions. He was also nationally well-known for his write-up on "Killer Stress" published in a leading magazine put up by a drug company, and a book on "45 Ways of Busting Stress," which became a popular seller.

The Psychiatrist is also a member of the Focolare movement, a religious organization. He is a strong advocate of "holistic healing" as one of the best forms of psychiatric management. He is a lifetime member of the YMCA.

Dr. "Lito," as he is called by love ones and friends, hails from Valencia, an inland town west of the provincial capital, Dumaguete City. The good doctor and his family have established residence in Dumaguete where he savors his retirement in full.

www.ingramcontent.com/pod-product-compliance
Lightning Source LLC
Chambersburg PA
CBHW032049020426
42335CB00011B/247